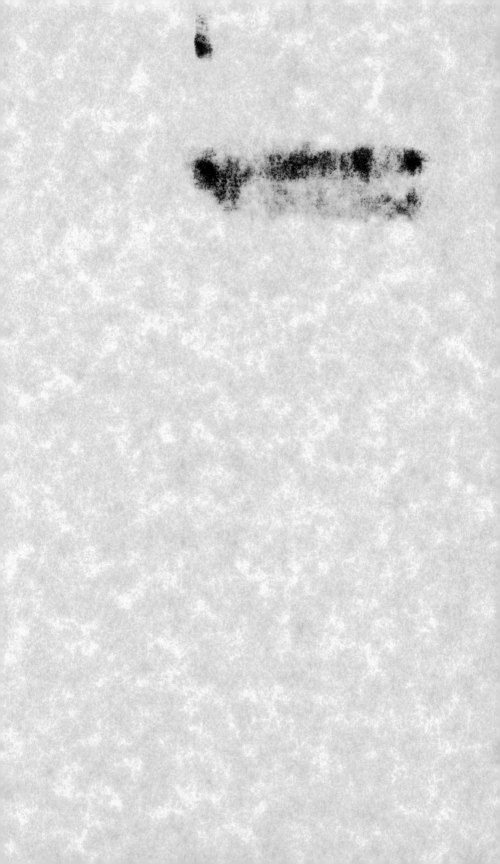

MEDICAL CARE OF THE SOUL

MEDICAL CARE
OF THE SOUL

A Practical & Healing Guide to
End-of-Life Issues for Families, Patients,
& Health Care Providers

Bruce G. Bartlow, MD

Chaplain ;
Michael Angelo Ongula

Johnson Books
BOULDER

Published in the United States by Johnson Books, a division of Johnson Publishing Company, 1880 South 57th Court, Boulder, Colorado 80301. E-mail: books@jpcolorado.com

9 8 7 6 5 4 3 2 1

Cover design by Debra B. Topping

Library of Congress Cataloging-in-Publication Data
Bartlow, Bruce G.
  Medical care of the soul: a practical and healing guide to end-of-life issues for families, patients, and health care providers / Bruce G. Bartlow.
      p.   cm.
  Includes bibliographical references and index.
  ISBN 1-55566-253-6 (alk. paper) — ISBN 1-55566-254-4 (p. alk. paper)
  1. Death—Handbooks, manuals, etc. 2. Terminally ill—Se   r. 3. Terminally ill—Care. I. Title.

GT3150 .B345 2000
306.9—dc21   00-029644

Printed in the United States by
Johnson Printing
1880 South 57th Court
Boulder, Colorado 80301

 Printed on recycled paper with soy ink

To Joshua and Maya,
the dearest of souls
and the best explanation I know
for life in the universe

Contents

Acknowledgments   IX

Part One: The Source
  1 When Death Changes Everything   3

Part Two: On Troubled Waters
  2 Arranging the Last of Your Life   15
  3 What Needs to Be Considered?   21
  4 Advance Directives and Other Confusions   27
  5 Who Needs to Participate, and How?   57
  6 Into the Darkness: Discussing the End of Life   75
  7 Finding the Way Home: Conflicts and
     Their Resolution   85

Part Three: A Stone in the River
  8 Technology, Slayer of the Soul: Our Struggle
     to Deny the Soul's Message   107
  9 When Society's Soul Speaks: Damning
     the Patient   123
 10 The Illusion of Cure: Hoping to Escape   139
 11 Shall We Do Everything ... or Nothing?   145
 12 The Descent: By the Road of Tears Will We
     Find Our Way to Healing   151

Part Four: The River Runs Through Us

13 Medical Care of the Soul 163
14 The Soul's Calling: Illness as the Way In 167
15 The Soul as Individual: I Will Pass This
Way Only Once 191
16 The Soul as Eternal Being: What I Came
Here to Learn 207
17 The Soul as Legacy: Beneath the Stones,
These Words 225
18 The Soul as Manifestation of the "One":
We All Come to Be Healed 243

Part Five: Completing the Journey

19 As I Lay Dying: Completing Life Through
Illness and Death 255
20 The Healer's Path 271

Bibliography 273
Source Notes 277
Index 279

Acknowledgments

As I begin this book, I must express my deepest gratitude to all those who have pushed me along this journey from naive reveries of omnipotence to the mysterious questions of our purpose on earth. I must first and most fervently thank all the patients and families who drew me into their lives in their darkest moments. I would include among the most poignant of these Jay Monaco and his children, Angie and A.J. They welcomed me into their hearts and the last of his life with a generosity that healed all of us. Even if I was too busy or dense to realize it at the time, they were my teachers one and all. I thank the nurses, doctors, therapists, housekeepers, clerks, and lab techs who often know so much more than I about my patients as human beings. I can't begin to count the times they've grabbed me by the shoulder and whispered, "Excuse me, but your patient was telling me that what she really needs just now is ..."

I thank all the community members who have participated in the evolution of these ideas through seminars and meetings. Most particularly, I thank the clergy who blessed me in the right direction and didn't string me up by my thumbs for writing about something like the soul, which is hereditarily their turf. I received patient, gentle, and amazingly wise guidance in Medical Ethics from Dr. Laurence Schneiderman of the University of California, San Diego; Dr. Ernlé Young of Stanford University; and Steve Heilig at the San Francisco Medical Society.

For the actual creation of this book, the list of mitzvahs must begin with Barbara Paley, who is really named Bobbi. She has believed in me and nudged me along for half a lifetime, apparently understanding how the world actually works. I received wonderfully tender editorial abuse from Christina Cicero of Redding, CA, and Jim Wade of Yorktown Heights, NY. Crucial review comments came from Ed Dundas, Valerie Springer, David Ermann, Marie Dodd, Jan Gandy, Katherine Garrison, Sharon Owen, Kay Morris-Long, and my brother Michael, who concluded, "If a person were to be looking for some deep thoughts, this book would be just the place to go."

Finally, and before all of this, from the other side of death's passage a beautiful, silver-haired lady with a pixie hairdo and clacking teeth smiles knowingly, chuckling at my chutzpah. Her name is Beatrice Tucker. She was an obstetrician for a hundred years, it seemed; one of those years she took a dazed young medical student by the scruff of his neck and taught him the beauties and tragedies of how life wrenches its way into the world. She taught me about the forever unfulfillable yearning a death interjects into the flow of life and the guilty insufficiency one feels at having neglected a dear one's irreplaceable soul. With typical generosity, she guides me even today. The best of this book is a testimony to the rich humanity she demonstrated to me, long before I was ready to receive it.

PART ONE

The Source

Eventually, all things merge into one, and a river runs through it. The river was cut by the world's great flood and runs over rocks from the basement of time. On some of the rocks are time-less raindrops. Under the rocks are the words, and some of the words are theirs.

I am haunted by waters.

—Norman Maclean,
A River Runs Through It

ONE

When Death
Changes Everything

*A*LL OF US WILL COME to the end of our lives, but so few of us will die well.

Nearly everyone who reads this book will someday care for a friend or family member as they die. Some of us will even make it a profession. Though we offer our help out of love, I believe we also hope to be nourished by the transcendent experience of participating in a life well lived and released with grace. Sadly, we're more likely to find ourselves wounded, drained to the core by the brutality of the last of life as it is acted out in our technologic world.

Thirty years of trying to "save" critically ill and dying patients have convinced me that this squandering, this disfigurement, of the last of life happens because we ignore the unfinished purposes our souls would pursue. When I speak of the soul, I mean that essential spark that most deeply defines each of us. You may experience it through your community of worship, through meditation or a quiet time in the woods. You may sense "soul" as the eternal or the profoundly intimate, the unique or the universal. But this much is certain: death in these modern times is considered to be nothing but loss and failure. We have forgotten how to hear that ancient voice within each of us, urging us to learn that we may heal and be healed.

The pages that follow tend to be in the language of the soul: metaphorical, poetic, often ambivalent. If we will listen to the

3

haunting music of illness and death, we will learn how to compose the meaning of our lives. Our intent should be not just to prolong a life but to honor Life as a cohesive work of informed beauty.

If we can learn to look at death as our souls see the conclusion of this life, we will discover in death a richly illuminating panorama of possibility, intrigue, and revealing mystery.

If we can learn to feel death as our souls experience death deep in our hearts, the terrified chill in our bones will be warmed by the love of those we hold most dear.

If we can learn to know death as a passing into the sheltering arms of our souls, we will find the strength to reshape our entire lives.

How shall we hear the clear call of this most essential part of our-selves through all the busy racket that makes up our daily lives? How can our souls make us pay attention? For many of us, it is only ill-ness or the approach of death that turn us toward the questions we were born to ask.

When the Waters Part

So many times we look in the mirror or catch our reflections in still water. Then one day we are startled to look back and discover either a spirit exuding a radiant clarity or a soiled skeleton stripped of all of life's once glowing promise. Usually we see both.

For each of us there is the moment when Death comes up from behind. He may stalk us or grab us by the throat or just walk many miles and years in our shadow. But we each know in some unspo-ken, indefinable way when he arrives. From then on, nothing will ever be the same.

The river of life seemed to be running so smoothly. Suddenly here is a stone that disrupts everything. The water goes murky and tur-bulent. The elements of time and change break our illusions of im-mortality. We sink into fear—How will what remains of my finite worldly existence play out? How will I be treated when I lose the power to determine my fate?

Out of control, drowning in emotions, we may encounter beneath the surface of life the love of those who for good or ill have shared our time here. If we are very lucky and choose very well indeed, we finally may reap the joys of crystal-clear understanding. It was an illness and the palpable reality of death, that stone in the river, that called me to take hold of the rest of my life before it was too late.

When Death Comes Calling, Close the Door!

All the busyness that our health care system piles up around the end of a life is an attempt to draw a thin veil over what we dread most: the fact that death waits for the families and health care providers as surely as for the patient being cared for at the moment. We watch our loved ones fade away, knowing that soon we will be next in line. Even those of us who work daily with the dying are totally unprepared; we haven't a clue as to the look or feel of this thing we've been wrestling our entire professional lives, and we ... are ... scared. It is this fear, not our vaunted professionalism or the pressures of time, that keeps us from exploring the wisdom our souls present to us through our final traumas. The transition out of life brings us to one of the three experiences we will share with every one of our patients: death, birth, and this brief life that connects them. Tragically, we trade these priceless moments for the delusion that life can be prolonged indefinitely.

Our society invests up to 30 percent of health care resources in "caring for" the last six months of life. What do we misunderstand that we make so costly an undertaking such a disaster?

Through my intense participation in the mess we make of the end of life, I've arrived at several conclusions that are the core of this book:

1. I have come to believe that our denial of the soul's calling is the wound that makes so much of medical care destructive, humiliating, and pointless. We take life's crises as an invading army of miserable inconveniences we must fight or suffer. In fact they are much

more: they are the soul's way of calling us to heal ancient wounds and learn new ways to be, to see, to touch and be touched. Part Two, "On Troubled Waters," looks at practical steps we can take to arrange the end of life and what roles each participant can play.

2. Much of our resources and energy are devoted to denying or evading the soul's call. We desperately apply technology in pursuit of a "cure," no matter what damage we may do in the process. Blame and judgment often affect which treatments we make available. We cut our world into opposites—doing "everything" or "nothing"—forcing ourselves into destructive choices. Part Three, "A Stone in the River," discusses the stages of denial, anger, and bargaining by which we finally arrive at "The Descent" into depression and hopelessness. It is there that we begin the work of the soul.

3. Illness and death are often the soul's last, desperate chance to be recognized and honored and to achieve its goals. Part Four, "The River Runs Through Us," looks at how we can hear the soul's call and come to know this soul that speaks to us through the story of our lives.

4. The illusion of separation between "patients" and "caregivers" prevents all of us from reaching for the wholeness our souls offer us at the end of a journey well traveled.

5. By envisioning our own deaths from the soul's perspective, each of us can transform what remains of this life. We can then live out for years all the lessons our deaths will someday try to teach us.

Look Out, Bro', Here Come de Vampire!

Death first made my acquaintance the summer of '67. It was three months before starting medical school. I was entering a medical facility for the first time since my birth. I felt small and very foreign as I approached the forbidding stone ramparts of Chicago Veterans' Hospital.

It was the sort of cheery Chicago dawn when muggers prowl behind every bush and the piles of garbage seem to take on their own life. My early arrival was occasioned by one of those nauseating ironies so typical of modern medicine: in this case, drawing blood in return for food. Over the next two years the predawn hours would find me coaxing samples from the battered vessels of alcoholics and drug addicts, heroic veterans, and whimpering wrecks—the best of men and so many who already had fully given up their best. In the shadowed rooms, row upon row of groggy patients braced themselves for my arrival. When I drew the "harpoons" from the pockets of my short white coat, the thick air filled with taunts of "Look out, bro', here come de vampire," and "Oh, shit, the new guy again."

Death probably became my companion too often during those years of my youth. In film clips from far away Vietnam, on the wards and outside in the dark alleys of the city, death constantly reminded me and my peers that we weren't necessarily in charge. Given their histories and the facilities available to us, my patients in Chicago didn't have a chance in hell. But the biggest problem I faced would be how not to crack my skull open when I fell asleep during the morning lecture.

Around me throbbed a vast medical juggernaut that exceeded in its marvels and contradictions anything I could have imagined. Medicine's techniques, pathways, pitfalls, and pratfalls were as hidden from me as the innermost chambers of the Great Pyramid of Gaza. Nevertheless, I knew with absolute certainty the purpose of the priesthood I was about to join: *We will save lives!*

Since then I've tried to decode the secrets of a million heartbeats as veritable rivers of blood passed through the many medical institutions in which I've worked. I've celebrated all the sacred rites of technologic medicine, from patching the lame to revitalizing the dead, from cutting to sewing to pasting. Like a good soldier in some vast European war, I've devoted my energies to fighting the endless pitched battles that modern medicine wages on the fields of our patients' bodies and spirits.

The taunts of those patients early in my career echo in my ears today. As individuals and as a society, we've begun to wonder whether medical care is a savior proffering vials of eternal youth or a vampire come to drain away our most vital resources.

Who Cares About Death?

This book is for all of us who are facing death or will someday die. We all will be there, but few of us admit it to ourselves. Our deaths almost certainly will occur in a hospital. The process is likely to be prolonged and unpleasant. We will feel at a loss, frightened, out of control. A 1995 study called SUPPORT (1) showed that death in American hospitals is a miserable business, seldom proceeding as the patient or family would wish. Worse, doctors have little idea of our patients' wishes or their families' needs. It gets even worse than that: when doctors in the study were informed of their patients' prognoses and concerns, there was no change in physician behavior or medical orders to reflect the patients' desires. The doctors either didn't listen or didn't consider the information relevant.

Why this deafening absence of communication? Listen to it closely: you'll hear the sounds of denial and confusion. When we truly admit the imminence or even the possibility of death, we uncover a potpourri of questions both urgent and eternal. As each of us battles, suffers, or finally yields, there comes the moment when we can ask, "What will I tolerate to achieve what possible benefit? What is the purpose that will justify my suffering?

"What do I fear, and what do I love? How do I face and ingest the enormity of these two conflicting emotions that ultimately encompass so much of human experience? How do I formulate the last of my life to honor all that went before and will be left behind? What do I need to complete now, while I can?

"What will I grieve? When will the grieving end?

"When did it begin? Why didn't I notice sooner?"

Many of us who haven't yet acknowledged our personal mortality are drawn into death's nagging presence because we are family members or friends of someone who is dying or will soon die. Odds are, we're going to be dissatisfied with how the last of our loved ones' lives play out in the medical system. In the hospital setting, we may well be treated like a bunch of troublesome, intruding outsiders. As I've presented this material at community conferences, it has become evident that the families have the hardest road to travel. Their roles are unclear, their pain and bewilderment seldom addressed. Their needs usually go unnoticed as everyone focuses on the patient and the medical procedures he or she requires. An illness may last a few months or a few days. But those who cared will carry the regrets and resentments of that final time for decades to come.

The questions facing family and friends are a bit different than those that confront the person who is dying at the moment: "Can we save him? How do we let him go, yet live with ourselves? What should we do? Where do we stand? When is it proper for me to go to the bathroom? Where in the devil is the bathroom, anyway?" Rarely are families guided from the physical procedures to the deeper purposes: What is unresolved? How do we begin to realize her legacy? How do we want to remember him at the end? How would she want to write the play of her final scene, to shape the stories that will live beyond her? How do we want to remember our participation in the last of her life?

And a particular subset of us, called health care providers, find ourselves immersed in questions having to do with the end of life because we have chosen to work with the seriously ill and dying. We tell ourselves we wish to cure or save others. This traditional understanding of our powers, limits, and proper goals is proving horribly inappropriate. Like a Vietnamese village wiped out in order to be liberated, our patients are often destroyed by the technologic brilliance we heap upon them. It is my sincere hope that this book will be part of a long-overdue sea change. I contend that we come not only to cure but also to be cured in return; we are limited not by our technology but by the paucity of our imagination and empathy.

As healers, our deepest and most urgent goals must be not just to maintain biologic survival but to unleash the potential of our patients' and our own souls. When we withdraw in confusion and fear from the most essential questions, we tend to lose touch with our most profound sources of sustaining wisdom—doubt, pain, personal experience, spiritual revelation, intimacy with those closest to us. We become drained rather than filled. Because we isolate our human vulnerability and need from the dramas around us, we end up feeling used rather than used well.

A Good Death

A very dear friend and Argentine physician, Ernesto Espinosa, tells of an inscription carved over the entrance to the Facultad de Medicina in Buenos Aires. As each medical student enters the cloistered realm of the school, the words they pass just overhead are, "El Trabajo del Médico Es No Solo Preservar la Salud, sino Ayudar a Bien Morir": in effect, "A Good Life, a Good Death." My colleagues and I, and most of us in the West, have forgotten that the Hippocratic commitment not to do harm may supersede our efforts to prolong physical life. Nor is responsibility to pursue healing limited to the needs of the body. We are under no mandate to maintain life no matter what the cost: if we force our patient to endure a life he or she would abhor, we do irreparable damage to our patient, the family, ourselves, and all of our souls. By embracing death's gifts, we will learn to revitalize the life of which the death is one small part. By envisioning well our own deaths, hours or perhaps years in advance, we will become able to explore fully the lives our souls came here to know.

The day came when I had pretty much finished this book. I'd written my way through denial into depression, filled out all the forms, and addressed the end of life. To my surprise, I found myself writing my own death, based on the principles that had fallen into place. With each honest word, each new paragraph, I felt my fears dissolving into love. Opening a door long closed, I discovered a joy that had waited a lifetime or more to be welcomed back into my consciousness. I was called to look deeply at what might have been different, back then, now, while I still have time.

Chapter 19, "As I Lay Dying," is this vision of my own death, based on the ideas that had evolved through writing the previous sections. When I experience such awareness, the hours or years remaining to me carry the lightness of celestial gifts. I'd recommend such an exploration to everyone as soon as you can possibly manage it. My deepest hope is that this book will help you find your way there.

That story begins, "So, now I am dying." Since we all are, then let it be for the good.

PART TWO

On Troubled Waters

*H*ope lies not only in an expectation of
cure or even of the remission of present
distress. For dying patients, the hope of cure will
always be shown to be ultimately false, and even
the hope of relief too often turns to ashes. When
my time comes, I will seek hope in the knowledge
that insofar as possible I will not be allowed to
suffer or be subjected to needless attempts to
maintain life; I will seek it in the certainty that I
will not be abandoned to die alone; I am seeking it
now, in the way I try to live my life, so that those
who value what I am will have profited by my time
on earth and be left with comforting recollections
of what we have meant to one another.

—Sherwin B. Nuland, *How We Die*

TWO

Arranging the Last
of Your Life

*M*Y FIRST TWENTY YEARS after medical school included
military medicine in Karlsruhe, Germany, desperate medicine during the Sudanese famine of 1984–1985, and the "heroic"
efforts of technologic medicine in half a dozen critical-care units. I
came to know what it is to face vast populations dying from totally
treatable causes while across the globe we might spend in one day
on one patient something approaching the entire health budget of
a huge African nation.

By August 1993 I had become director of St. Luke's Subacute
Unit in San Francisco. It was my responsibility to throw vast mountains of resources at patients in coma or permanently on ventilators.
As each patient was carted into the unit, I would ask his or her family members why they had chosen such treatment for their loved
one. The answers ran something like this: "We were never asked";
"They said we had to do this or it would be murder"; or the ever popular and usually irate "Of course we have to keep him alive. We can't
just do nothing."

I was also directing the Intensive Care Unit (ICU), where 30 percent of all hospital expenditures go to those patients least likely to
survive. The third aspect of my career was as a kidney specialist man-
aging patients on dialysis. Approaching my twentieth year as a
nephrologist, I watched more and more of my dialysis patients sink

into existences that seemed to me to be nothing but pure misery. On the rare occasions when I asked a patient what he was getting in return for his and our trouble, he usually would look at me through gaunt eyes and ask, "Well, what's the alternative?"

I voiced my disillusionment about the evil I was doing to my patients in an editorial in the *San Francisco Chronicle*. I blamed the horrifying fruits of our technology on the cult of individual rights without responsibilities. I suggested that one day we must consider the possibility that different lives have different worth, that a year of life in a vegetative state (perpetual coma) may not be worth more than vaccinating ten thousand children. A patient suffering on a ventilator but unable to demand release might not consider her life worth the entire health care costs for one hundred families. (The editors cut out the suggestion that the insurance CEO's work is not worth $118,000,000 when a nurse makes $20,000, or that a physician may not be justified in making oodles of loot keeping the unsalvageable alive just because the "standard of care" involves always doing the most, not the best. It always struck me as significant that those were the sections the paper saw fit *not* to print.)

Then I hunkered down and got ready for the slaughter. I had gored the sacred bull of every American's right to all he or she can get. I was sure the ferocious backlash would prove my daring.

To my utter astonishment, *ninety* community members and health care providers wrote in heartfelt agreement. Nurses had abandoned long, devoted careers because an administrator or supervisor had censured them for discussing the possibility of withdrawing technologic life support. Decades after a loved one had died, families were still grieving or enraged over how the last of life had been twisted by the health care providers, with the family members' acquiescence. Other families and friends lived in horrible guilt because they had consented to have such abuses perpetrated on those they had meant to protect. Patients and spouses wrote, asking for a way to protect themselves from such disasters. Dozens of people were bewildered that our society could waste so many resources and cause so much

pointless pain, all for two lovely but intrinsically insane notions—
that life can be prolonged endlessly and that the cost in dollars and
suffering is irrelevant.

I didn't get off unscathed. Two kidney specialists' letters howled,
"You idiot, you're trying to put us out of business!" One physician
and two nurses said, "We have to do this or we'll get sued!" One re-
spondent at that time, and two in magazines since, accused me of
advocating something close to Nazi eugenics: this jackbooted, self-
righteous Dr. Bartlow would abandon entire classes of people—the
elderly, disabled, gay, HIV positive, poor—because someone would
decide they weren't good enough. Such is our fear: if we admit there
is any difference between two individuals, we'll start shipping people off to the ovens.

The fact is, we all teeter on the slippery slope. No two of us give
the same value to our lives, our goals, our suffering, our outcomes.
No two of us want the same things. No two of us see the world the
same way. Even if we could, no two of us would write our story the
same way beneath the stones of time.

How can each of us identify and enunciate the views that are
uniquely our own in a way that will prove clear, relevant, and binding? How can we be assured that these views will be heard and
honored?

If I'm to make the best use of my remaining time, I must first acknowledge that I will die. I must grasp in my own two hands the opportunity to review my life and plan its completion. When I declare
how I choose to be, I establish my individual Constitution. When I
define what treatment I will or will not accept, I create my own Bill
of Rights. I can determine who will decide for me when I become
unable to do so myself. Which burdens do I accept? What outcome
would I find worthwhile? How is my body to be handled? At what
point should this shell I carry around be abandoned, written off,
plowed under? To whom should my remains be handed?

Once I realize that I can actively envision and shape the last
stages of my life, I will require certain tools. I must become aware of

what *questions* are pertinent. I will require a valid and clear way of *communicating* my thoughts. I must consider *who* should participate in such decisions, and *how*. Taking a deep breath, I must be willing to plunge into a discussion of my *values, hopes, and fears*. When the inevitable conflicts and confusions arise, I need a structured way to *resolve* them. The conflicts we face are not just between patients and doctors. They're between me and various members of my family, be-tween my illusions and my reality, between who I've been and who my soul declares I was meant to be and can still become.

These conflicts are in fact not just troublesome stumbling blocks. They are the best window we have on what we need to heal before death concludes our journey through this lifetime.

I could make a good living betting that those of you reading this book have never had such discussions. My colleagues typically offer four reasons for not addressing end-of-life decisions with our pa-tients. These are:

1. My patients wouldn't want to hear about such frightening stuff.
2. I don't have time.
3. I know what she wants.
4. It's not my role to initiate such discussions.

The real story beneath the spoken words is:

1. I'm uncomfortable mentioning death.
2. I don't know how to broach these issues.
3. Fact is, I don't really even know what the issues are.
4. Hell no, I won't go there.

This section includes discussions that families, patients, and health care providers will need to shape the rest of our lives. "In the beginning was the Word." By the words we write and communicate, we each become our own God-Creator. If we face the last of our lives with silent denial, we will see only a terrifying abyss. If we approach the last of our time here as we would a soul mate we've sought since before birth, we will fill the remaining hours or years with tender, illuminating passion. Through the words and touch we offer those who are near us as we live and inevitably die, we begin to establish the legacy of how we have lived and will live on forever. Cardinal Bernadin, dying of cancer, saw not an enemy but a friend in death. By welcoming and writing about that sense of comfort, he expanded death's circle of friendship to thousands, perhaps millions of other souls.

How do we begin the discussion of end-of-life decisions? Imagine sitting down in an examining room or consultation area, or perhaps on a hospital bed in the midst of a crisis. You may be a patient, a family member, or friend. Perhaps you're a health care provider preparing to discuss some near stranger's desires for arranging the last of a long life.

Some words are exchanged, some forms change hands, but something much more profound has been called into the room. That which is most human in us is deeply touched by another and draws us toward trusting introspection. The participants in the discussion feel suddenly not alone.

Each of us, seeing someone find strength and direction as they meet death, may experience the first glimmer of reassurance that our powers will not end when our health, our life, begin slipping away. Nor will we lose our power when we can no longer speak, nor when our breath ceases; not even when we are physically gone. Our actions and words, if shared with a courageous clarity, will achieve everything we're ready to complete.

The family members or friends in the room begin to see how much they have to offer and how much to learn from this loved one in their final times together. And the physician, nurse, or counselor may be reminded that we came to this work not just to keep pasting bodies together but to experience some deep mystery in ourselves and those for whom we care. Our greatest power will be as fellow travelers on this scary yet startlingly beautiful adventure.

THREE

What Needs to Be Considered?

C URRENT DISCUSSIONS OF end-of-life issues range from nothing (in 90 percent of cases) to a series of questions involving
interventions, timing, and what to do if the results fall short of some
ill-defined "acceptable" outcome. What characterizes virtually all of
these discussions is that they tend to focus on *procedures* and yes-or-
no decisions.

In planning the end of a life, this approach is further complicated
by the unknowable: What illness or trick of fate might bring me to
a point where I couldn't express my wishes and might require cardiopulmonary resuscitation (CPR) in order to survive? The apparently
simple decision of whether or not to resuscitate may become either
ridiculously complex or utterly arbitrary. For example, a healthy
thirty-four-year-old man with HIV (AIDS virus) has seen too many
of his friends die long, anguished deaths. He completes a "Do Not Resuscitate" (DNR) Advance Directive. One day, crossing the street, he's
hit by a truck. He would recover completely in a few days, but the
injury to his lung requires a ventilator, which his DNR precludes.
Should I let him die of an unforeseen, totally reversible problem?

Or let's say a sixty-eight-year-old woman demands that "all efforts
be made to prolong my life, regardless of my chances of recovery."
A year later she has become demented, unable to care for herself,
and incontinent of urine and stool. Her family members feel she

would have hated living in such a condition. Although her Advance Directive spoke of *procedures*, it's the *quality of her life* that is at issue. How long does her Advance Directive require me to prolong her humiliation?

If we are to begin our journey toward the soul, toward the most essential parts of each individual, we must begin with how we value our lives. What is an acceptable quality of existence? Which burdens are acceptable for which outcomes? What constitutes an undue burden?

Again, I would respond to the physician who complains, "I don't have time for such elaborate discussions," by being very clear: these concerns are so vital to each of us, and so deeply held, that we don't require a great deal of time to begin the discussion. What begins as a fearful attempt to limit bodily harm quickly becomes an exploration shared between the patient and his or her family and friends that will reveal the soul's needs and hopes for the last of life. Time is never really the issue in caregivers' refusal to discuss wishes for the end of life: the real reason is our denial of death and our discomfort with the great mysteries we've never considered. I've found that our approach needs to be virtually the reverse of that usually taken: tell me what you hope to achieve, and I'll tell you whether my procedures can buy you enough time and energy to get there.

We should begin with **Goals:** What do you hope to learn or heal by the end of this illness and its treatment? Is it biologic survival that matters, or making it to Christmas? Might you encourage your children to stop fighting and love one another again? Do you just plain want to cost society as much as you can in order to make up for everything you were cheated out of in the course of a long and hard life? Was there a dream you always held dear? If so, can you achieve it now?

What is your soul seeking to understand about itself through this illness?

Hopes for the remainder of life: What is unresolved; what needs to be mended; what needs to be released? What legacy do you want to leave behind you? What level of functioning will you need if you're to achieve your goals? What intolerable pain or sadness do you hope can be eased as this illness passes through you?

What does your soul hope to learn by the end of this illness or this lifetime?

Fears: What outcome or symptoms do you most dread? Is your worst nightmare that you may become disabled or disfigured? Does dependency or abandonment, pain, nausea, or itching scare you most? Is it uncertainty? Is it loss of control, or never being able to give up the control? Do you dread consuming your family's emotional or material resources so that you leave only a legacy of despair and destitution?

What you most fear may be what your soul has brought you to this point to face, to experience, and to accept. The most terrifying, emptiest spot within us may be exactly where our soul waits. Perhaps only by losing what we thought we couldn't live without can we find grace and peace.

Quality of life, before and after the illness or interventions: Is your present quality of life one you wish to continue? If not, what needs to be changed? What quality of life would you find acceptable after the illness or procedures? What do you want us to do if we can't achieve that outcome for you?

This question gives your soul the chance to be heard and makes many of life's frustrations and joys fit into an understandable pattern. Can you use this opportunity to reconcile your inner and outer lives? What made you set up such contradictions between what you live and what you feel you could be? What powers, what yearnings does this illness give you the chance to explore in yourself and in those you cherish or avoid?

Clinical situation (or hypothetical situation in Advance Directives): What are you facing? What is the likely impact of this illness and the proposed procedures on your life afterward? What can you reasonably hope for, and what should you fear? At what level are you threatened—survival? loss? limitation? And how—emotionally? spiritually? financially?

If you watch closely, you can sense your soul hovering just over your shoulder, watching, studying you, waiting to see how you'll react to this new challenge. You can feel your soul tightening muscles in some part of you—one or many of the energy levels I'll mention in the last chapter of this section.

Burdens of the proposed interventions: What risks and discomforts do the procedures entail? Are there other procedures less damaging? What risks would you find most onerous? What outcomes deemed "successful" by your health care providers would you find too burdensome? How much does the therapy cost in dollars, inconvenience, and risk, and who's going to pay the price? What suffering is involved, not just at the level of physical pain but at the levels of emotion, self-image, and spirit? How much will you hurt? How much will it change how you feel about yourself as you look in the mirror or remember what you went through? Will a "heroic" intervention add to your sense of the world as a place of love and safety or as a place of violence and indifference to you as a precious being?

Ask yourself if the burdens imposed by the intervention will lead you deeper into what your soul needs to explore or will in fact so distract or incapacitate you that you'll not be able to complete your soul's work.

Likely benefits: These are all we usually consider—"Here, just let us whip your gallbladder out and you'll be all better. We'll put new pipes in your heart and you'll be able to charge back into a life of smoking, swearing, and eating fat for another couple of years." But how likely is the best outcome, and how likely the worst?

CPR provides a particularly stark example of the need to explore goals and likely benefits. The fact that we do it to everyone unless specifically ordered otherwise suggests that it's a greatly beneficial procedure. When asked, health care providers consistently estimate the chance of a successful outcome from CPR at roughly three times the real figure. Some representative statistics are:

Overall "success" of CPR (restoring pulse and respiration): 15 percent.

CPR "success" for patients over seventy years of age: 8 percent. *However,* only 2 percent survive to leave the hospital in a functional condition.

CPR for overwhelming pneumonia in the face of blood infection, liver failure, hematological malignancy such as leukemia, or kidney failure: 0 percent survive.

For patients over seventy years of age, CPR for less than five minutes for an abnormal heart rhythm: 60 percent survive. For longer than five minutes: 2 percent survive.

Children: 8 percent survive. Elderly people who were self-sufficient: 15 percent survive. Elderly people who required assistance for a variety of daily chores: 3 percent survive.

In other words, age, self-sufficiency, underlying conditions, cause of cardiopulmonary collapse, and the criterion used for "success" all affect our outlook. Since there's such a wide divergence between "successful" CPR and leaving the hospital alive, we would do well to address the quality of life post-CPR as opposed to mere biologic survival.

If there's anything the tragedy of the last of life in our medical system has shown, it's that there is a tremendous difference between "doing everything" and "doing everything appropriate." Will the intervention in fact permit you to fulfill your goals for what remains of your life? If not, is it time to change the goals, or time to change the proposed intervention?

If we focused on caring for our soul's needs rather than on a cure that would let us escape the illness's message, the greatest benefit of all would accrue: our lives themselves might be ordered anew. Our appreciation of the life we've lived might be transformed. The meaning of our personal drama might become clear.

Finding the soul by filling out the next chapter's forms about your desires for the end of life is a peculiar business. It's a bit like looking just to the side of someone to catch their spirit out of the corner of your eye, or coming up with a great insight while you're raking leaves. These issues of death, danger, and the end of one's individual "time" may evoke parts of your mind and spirit that have been trying to come through for as long as you've been on earth. Listen to them if they speak up. When you notice them, at the margins of your field of vision, turn toward them rather than away.

FOUR

Advance Directives and Other Confusions

W E ARE A LITERATE PEOPLE, with an inordinate trust in written words. Medicine's governing board, the Joint Commission on Accreditation of Healthcare Organizations, determines caregivers' suitability to touch human beings based on documentation.

As patients and as health care providers, our documents both serve and determine us. We confuse checking a box on a paper with making a clear and accurate statement of our wishes. The forms that have been developed to format end-of-life discussions therefore take on an aura of incredible power. We medical professionals will give more credence to a check mark on an Advance Directive (AD) than to the spouse who has lived sixty years with our patient. She will be at his bedside through all the days and long, grueling nights of the upcoming trauma and will live with the consequences of what we do. Yet we send the family away at the crucial moment to find us the piece of paper we naively believe will make everything clear.

The Questions to Ask

As you review the various Advance Directive forms I've included at the end of this chapter, there are certain questions you need to ask yourself about each format. These include:

- When will the forms apply?
- Who knows what you really intend to express? Who needs to know?
- Does the paper say what you think it says?
- What are the opportunities for misunderstanding?
- Where will you put the piece of paper so it can be found when it is needed?
- What important aspects of the last of your life are *not* addressed by this document?
- Therefore, what other explanations do you need to make?
- In filling out this document, and in the discussions that ensued, what other questions or issues did you discover you need to pursue now, while there's still time, today?

I would also reiterate the questions I feel every Directive must address if it's to guide medical decisions to your soul's purpose. These are:

- Goals
- Hopes
- Fears
- Quality of life before and after the illness
- Clinical situation you're envisioning
- Burdens of therapy proposed (for instance, CPR)
- Benefits of therapy you'd find acceptable (for instance, survival versus function)

The Documents

There are several general categories of document, each with certain strengths and liabilities. Some have been generated by lawyers, some by concerned citizens, some by doctors (my own contribution to the evolutionary process is included as "My Desires for the Last of My Life"), and some by multidisciplinary groups hoping to give form to essentially open-ended and unpredictable circumstances. The various approaches can be divided as follows:

1. The *"Durable Power of Attorney for Health Care Decisions"* designates who will speak for you but does little to express your own views. The catch here is that surrogates, that is, those asked to speak for you, in most cases haven't a clue what you want while at the same time suffering the tremendous emotional impact of their own love for you and their fears of failing you. Without discussions well in advance between you and your surrogates, they're shooting blind, likely to wound both you and themselves. It's noteworthy that when patients who have designated a surrogate are asked, "Who should decide if you can't?" only a third say their surrogate. Another third would place the power in the hands of their doctor, and the last third would designate their extended family or some other group.

The "Statement of Preferences" offers a box to check that your physician may interpret as "Do Everything" or "Do Nothing." Unless you can figure a way to state your values and the weight you give to different qualities of life and different burdens of therapy, suffering or survival, function or dependency, this box dooms your caregivers to utter confusion. The "Quality of Life" forms mentioned below are some of the attempts that have been made to clarify these very personal issues.

2. *"The California Living Will"* and *"Natural Death Act"* are examples of a patient's *binding* refusal of technologic intervention in relatively rare and strictly defined circumstances—terminal illness or irreversible coma. The question is, what is terminal—how soon, and what about quality of life in the meantime? And how sure do my doctors have to be that the coma is irreversible? What if I'm having a jolly old time in my terminal condition? Will the form rule if my family can't conceive of my thoroughly comatose body not remaining visibly in their world?

The *"Out of Hospital DNR (Do Not Resuscitate)"* is a similarly binding refusal of resuscitation by emergency workers. Unfortunately, it doesn't differentiate between reversible problems you might not anticipate (choking on a piece of steak) and terminal conditions in which resuscitation would either fail or only prolong suffering.

3. *"Quality of Life Advance Directives"*: Madlyn Brod's document describes several possible interventions and offers hypothetical situations for the patient and surrogate to consider together. It speaks to the questions of surrogacy and procedure, quality of life, and burden of therapy in a variety of possible circumstances.

I've developed a form that I titled, *"My Desires for the Last of My Life."* It expands on questions about quality of life, reversibility, suffering, goals, and who should decide. I believe this format most nearly approximates the discussions necessary to address the soul's desires.

4. *"Dying Well"*: I've included two pages from a twelve-month symposium designed for work groups by Ken Meese at St. Joseph's Hospital in Arcata, CA. The series was designed to make caregivers more aware of what is a good or bad death, what institutional structures foster one or the other, and what the person filling out the form would want for himself when he got down to the work of dying.

These forms have proven invaluable for patients and their families. In many cases they have been included as crucial adjuncts to the Advance Directive and even as the written legacy of a unique individual who passed our way and will long be remembered.

5. *"Five Wishes,"* by the Florida group Commission on Aging with Dignity, has achieved tremendous popularity on the East Coast. It does the most thorough job I've seen of focusing on goals, hopes, wishes, desires for yourself and your family, spiritual aspirations, the setting of the last of life, and guiding you to consider what you need to complete.

In all cases, the real value of whichever forms you choose lies not in the paperwork but in the discussions you have with your family, friends, caregivers, physicians, and nurses. No paper can capture all the desires, fears, and values of your soul. But each form raises important questions, the answers to which will be different for each person. The forms offer a means to explore your feelings and hopes. They give you the opportunity of leaving your family a final gift of peace and understanding. If done properly, they can protect you from unwanted interventions and your family from unnecessary guilt or anguish. But perhaps most importantly, they can direct you toward the questions we spend our lives avoiding: What did I come here to do? How do I want to prepare for what follows this life? How do I want to be remembered? What do I want to leave in the world? What delusions, bitterness, negativity am I finally ready to let go? What will be my true legacy? What did my soul come here to learn, and what will my soul take with it into the life I am about to be delivered into by my death?

When you define how you want the last of your life to evolve, thereby relieving your family of the burden of decision, you're creating a very important part of your legacy.

When you describe how much of a burden you would feel particular therapies to be, and what quality of life you would find acceptable, you're honoring your uniqueness as an individual.

When you define what experiences you hope to have or avoid at the end, you're arranging the last lessons your eternal being will take with it to what follows.

When we discuss these forms with those closest to us, we all experience ourselves as manifestations of the *One*. We all will face death. We all have the opportunity to create the best possible ends to our lives.

Tables 4.1–4.3 list these various AD styles with their strengths and weaknesses. These forms have little value unless you discuss them with your family, friends, and physicians. Which procedures are appropriate will depend greatly on whether they are likely to achieve a quality of life you would appreciate or cause a burden you would find intolerable. The alternative equation is the burden of disability or death imposed by not pursuing a given therapy.

Ideally, skilled practitioners would guide each of us through the procedural and "soul" questions. Unfortunately, one of my core motivations for writing this book was the utter lack of training we health care providers receive in how to approach such issues. We can help our patients and their families with the "technobabble,"

TABLE 4.1 Advance Directive Intents, Strengths, and Weaknesses

Form	Intent	Strengths	Weaknesses
"Durable Power"	Assigns surrogate. Defines wishes for life support.	Clarifies who will speak for the patient.	Surrogates seldom know patient's wishes.
	Legally tested.	Alludes to "burden versus benefit" and "quality of survival."	Doesn't define patient's values. Meaningless without these.
"Natural Death Act"	Demands DNR if terminal or comatose.	Clear and binding.	Very narrow circumstance. How soon terminal? How impaired?
"Quality of Life Advance Directive"	Defines patient's values for burden, quality of life, and relationship of procedures to likely outcomes.	Necessary to honor all of the above ADs; explores issues of soul, uniqueness, and legacy.	Hard to define all situations; requires discussion. "Qualitative" versus "quantitative," less clear, not legally tested.
"Dying Well"	Defines how the patient wishes to be treated.	Subjective and open.	No clear guidelines.
"Wishes"	Expresses patients' wishes for themselves, family, provider, caregivers.	Expands beyond procedures and the individual. Focuses on goals, legacy, and the exact scene of the end of life.	Very open ended, it may neglect specific procedures, reversibility, intermediate situations.

TABLE 4.2 Advance Directive Applications and Clarity

Form	Binding	When does it apply?	Clear about procedure	values	goals
"Durable Power"	to surrogate only	unable to speak for yourself	no	no	no
"Natural Death Act"	yes	terminal or comatose	yes	yes	no
"Quality of Life"	yes	variety of illnesses and procedures	yes	yes	a bit
"Dying Well"	no	anytime	possibly	yes	yes
"Wishes"	no	anytime	no	some	yes

TABLE 4.3 Applicability of Various Advance Directive Styles to the "Soul" Questions

Question	"Durable Power"	"Natural Death Act"	"Quality of Life"	"Dying Well"	"Wishes"
Goals	no	no	possibly	yes	yes
Hopes	no	no	possibly	yes	yes
Fears	yes	no	possibly	yes	yes
Quality of life	possibly	yes	yes	possibly	yes
Clinical situation	possibly	yes	possibly	possibly	yes
Burdens of therapy	possibly	no	yes	yes	yes
Benefits of therapy	possibly	no	possibly	possibly	yes

some of the realities of cardiopulmonary resuscitation and other procedures, and a mumbled reference to the alternatives to technologic
intervention. But at this point in the history of medicine, our patients may have more to teach us about achieving the deep values
of the last of life than we can ever begin to offer them in return.

The illness, decisions, and interventions and the iatrogenic illnesses created by the procedures we choose all challenge our spirits
and open opportunities for our souls' experience. We may learn more
from how we choose and why than from *what* we decide. Begin with
the form; end with a life-enhancing journey deeper into yourself.
Talk. Listen. Feel the caring and the hope that come from a dialog
with yourself and with those you love.

Whom to Contact for Additional Forms or Information

Your physician, hospital, lawyer, social worker or religious leader
Friends who've been through such decisions
Your state or local medical society
Choice in Dying, 200 Varick Street, New York, NY 10014-4810,
    212-366-5540
Center to Improve Care of the Dying, George Washington Univer-
    sity, 1001 22nd St. NW, Suite 820, Washington, DC, 20037, 202-
    467-2222
Hospice Association of America, 519 C Street NE, Washington, DC
    20002, 202-546-3540
National Family Caregivers Association, 9621 East Bexhill Drive,
    Kensington, MD 20895-3104, 301-942-6430
American Geriatrics Society, 770 Lexington Ave., Suite 300, New
    York, NY 10021, 212-308-1414
Midwest Bioethics Center, 1100 Pennsylvania Ave, Suite 4041,
    Kansas City, MO 64105, 816-221-2002
Commission on Aging with Dignity, PO Box 11180, Tallahassee, FL
    32302-1180, 888-5-WISHES

Advance Directive Forms (See pages 37–56)

"Durable Power of Attorney for Health Care Decisions" (Form 4.1)

This form designates a surrogate to speak for you when you cannot speak for yourself. It offers the chance to check off a box instructing caregivers *not* to prolong life in certain situations (undue burden, terminal illness, irreversible coma).

However, it doesn't clearly define what weight you give to specific burdens or value to specific outcomes. It also provides two (*only two!*) lines to write in your own wishes.

If you truly wish no technologic support, you have to write that in.

"Natural Death Act" (Form 4.2 A and B)

A. The "Directive to Physicians" absolutely refuses prolongation of life in two very specific and rare instances: terminal illness and irreversible coma.

B. The "Prehospital DNR" absolutely refuses resuscitation by emergency workers. However, it doesn't specify whether they should consider the reversibility of a problem in deciding whether to resuscitate, so you could die of an unanticipated, totally correctable problem.

"Quality of Life" (Form 4.3)

"Center for Clinical Aging Services Research": This double-sided document first hypothesizes a variety of clinical situations and asks which procedure you would want in each case. The second side describes various interventions that might be applied to prolong life.

This form relates procedures to quality of life *before* the intervention. The complexity of the grid befuddles many patients and leaves many situations uncovered.

"My Desires for the Last of My Life" (Form 4.4)

This form is my attempt to simplify the approach and add three additional issues: (1) reversibility, (2) goals through an illness or the last of life, and (3) desires for surrogacy.

"Dying Well" (Form 4.5)

These forms are a small part of a twelve-month exploration developed by Ken Meese for work groups in health care institutions. The two pages presented here offer the chance to answer two questions:

1. What qualities do you feel would characterize a good versus a bad death?
2. What hopes, needs, or requests do you have for yourself, your family, your providers, your environment, and others as you approach your death?

This form draws our attention toward the *bidirectional* nature of interactions at the end of life: what you hope to receive from and what you hope to give to those involved in the last of your life.

"Wishes" (Form 4.6)

"Five Wishes," from the Commission on Aging with Dignity, focuses on your desires for yourself, your family, your community, and your legacy. It gives considerable guidance toward arranging the last of your life.

California Medical Association
DURABLE POWER OF ATTORNEY FOR HEALTH CARE DECISIONS
(California Probate Code Sections 4600-4753)

WARNING TO PERSON EXECUTING THIS DOCUMENT

This is an important legal document. Before executing this document, you should know these important facts:

This document gives the person you designate as your agent (the attorney-in-fact) the power to make health care decisions for you. Your agent must act consistently with your desires as stated in this document or otherwise made known.

Except as you otherwise specify in this document, this document gives your agent power to consent to your doctor not giving treatment or stopping treatment necessary to keep you alive.

Notwithstanding this document, you have the right to make medical and other health care decisions for yourself so long as you can give informed consent with respect to the particular decision. In addition, no treatment may be given to you over your objection, and health care necessary to keep you alive may not be stopped or withheld if you object at the time.

This document gives your agent authority to consent, to refuse to consent, or to withdraw consent to any care, treatment, service, or procedure to maintain, diagnose, or treat a physical or mental condition. This power is subject to any statement of your desires and any limitations that you include in this document. You may state in this document any types of treatment that you do not desire. In addition, a court can take away the power of your agent to make health care decisions for you if your agent (1) authorizes anything that is illegal, (2) acts contrary to your known desires or (3) where your desires are not known, does anything that is clearly contrary to your best interests.

This power will exist for an indefinite period of time unless you limit its duration in this document.

You have the right to revoke the authority of your agent by notifying your agent or your treating doctor, hospital, or other health care provider orally or in writing of the revocation.

Your agent has the right to examine your medical records and to consent to their disclosure unless you limit this right in this document.

Unless you otherwise specify in this document, this document gives your agent the power after you die to (1) authorize an autopsy, (2) donate your body or parts thereof for transplant or therapeutic or educational or scientific purposes, and (3) direct the disposition of your remains.

If there is anything in this document that you do not understand, you should ask a lawyer to explain it to you.

1. CREATION OF DURABLE POWER OF ATTORNEY FOR HEALTH CARE

By this document I intend to create a durable power of attorney by appointing the person designated below to make health care decisions for me as allowed by Sections 4600 to 4753, inclusive, of the California Probate Code. This power of attorney shall not be affected by my subsequent incapacity. I hereby revoke any prior durable power of attorney for health care. I am a California resident who is at least 18 years old, of sound mind, and acting of my own free will.

2. APPOINTMENT OF HEALTH CARE AGENT

(Fill in below the name, address and telephone number of the person you wish to make health care decisions for you if you become incapacitated. You should make sure that this person agrees to accept this responsibility. The following may not serve as your agent: (1) your treating health care provider; (2) an operator of a community care facility or residential care facility for the elderly; or (3) an employee of your treating health care provider, a community care facility, or a residential care facility for the elderly, unless that employee is related to you by blood, marriage or adoption, or unless you are also an employee of the same treating provider or facility. If you are a conservatee under the Lanterman-Petris-Short Act (the law governing involuntary commitment to a mental health facility) and you wish to appoint your conservator as your agent, you must consult a lawyer, who must sign and attach a special declaration for this document to be valid.)

I, _____ , hereby appoint:
    (insert your name)

Name _____

Address _____

Work Telephone (_____) _____   Home Telephone (_____) _____

as my agent (attorney-in-fact) to make health care decisions for me as authorized in this document. I understand that this power of attorney will be effective for an indefinite period of time unless I revoke it or limit its duration below.

(Optional) This power of attorney shall expire on the following date: _____ .

3. AUTHORITY OF AGENT

If I become incapable of giving informed consent to health care decisions, I grant my agent full power and authority to make those decision for me, subject to any statements of desires or limitations set forth below. Unless I have limited my agent's authority in this document, th authority shall include the right to consent, refuse consent, or withdraw consent to any medical care, treatment, service, or procedure; receive and to consent to the release of medical information; to authorize an autopsy to determine the cause of my death; to make a gift of a or part of my body; and to direct the disposition of my remains, subject to any instructions I have given in a written contract for funer services, my will or by some other method. I understand that, by law, my agent may <u>not</u> consent to any of the following: commitment to mental health treatment facility, convulsive treatment, psychosurgery, sterilization or abortion.

4. MEDICAL TREATMENT DESIRES AND LIMITATIONS (OPTIONAL)

(Your agent must make health care decisions that are consistent with your known desires. You may, but are not required to, sta your desires about the kinds of medical care you do or do not want to receive, including your desires concerning life support if yo are seriously ill. If you do not want your agent to have the authority to make certain decisions, you must write a statement to th effect in the space provided below; otherwise, your agent will have the broad powers to make health care decisions for you that a outlined in paragraph 3 above. In either case, it is important that you discuss your health care desires with the person you appoi as your agent and with your doctor(s).

(Following is a general statement about withholding and removal of life-sustaining treatment. If the statement accurately reflec your desires, you may initial it. If you wish to add to it or to write your own statement instead, you may do so in the space provided.

I do **not** want efforts made to prolong my life and I do **not** want life-sustaining treatment to be provided or continued: (1) if I am in an irreversible coma or persistent vegetative state; or (2) if I am terminally ill and the use of life-sustaining procedures would serve only to artificially delay the moment of my death; or (3) under any other circumstances where the burdens of the treatment outweigh the expected benefits. In making decisions about life-sustaining treatment under provision (3) above, I want my agent to consider the relief of suffering and the quality of my life, as well as the extent of the possible prolongation of my life.

If this statement reflects your desires, initial here? _____

Other or additional statements of medical treatment desires and limitations: _____

_____

_____

_____

(You may attach additional pages if you need more space to complete your statements. Each additional page must be dated an signed at the same time you date and sign this document.)

5. APPOINTMENT OF ALTERNATE AGENTS (OPTIONAL)

(You may appoint alternate agents to make health care decisions for you in case the person you appointed in Paragraph 2 is unabl or unwilling to do so.)

If the person named as my agent in Paragraph 2 is not available or willing to make health care decisions for me as authorized in thi document, I appoint the following persons to do so, listed in the order they should be asked:

First Alternate Agent: Name _____

Address _____

Work Telephone (_____) _____   Home Telephone (_____) _____

Second Alternate Agent: Name _____

Address _____

Work Telephone (_____) _____   Home Telephone (_____) _____

6. USE OF COPIES

I hereby authorize that photocopies of this document can be relied upon by my agent and others as though they were originals.

FIVE

Who Needs to Participate, and How?

O UR SOCIETY'S narrow focus on the individual means that decisions about end-of-life care seem to involve only one person: the one whose life is being considered. That person checks the box, writes his or her unique wishes in his or her own hand, signs the thing before a witness, and hangs it on the refrigerator for the 911 crew to see. Whether anyone will notice it or know how to interpret it when the time comes is another issue altogether.

Legally and in our biomedical ethics, this absolute focus on the individual is a given. But I've come to believe that the true process is closer to a drama with perhaps half a dozen or more actors playing different and sometimes shifting roles. They all have their own ethnic, cultural, experiential, and philosophical baggage. They're at different points in the stories of their own lives. They're headed different directions and often seem stuck to a web in uncomfortable postures they can't escape. But they're all there, and they're all suddenly, unexpectedly, simultaneously forced into relationship.

It's not just one life that is ending. That individual's life is slipping away from all of the actors, just as they realize their own lives will one day end. A family and a web of friendships is about to be irrevocably altered. From now to the end of their lives, every survivor will be different from what they were before this illness and death came upon them.

57

We have to be clear first, about who the players are, and second, about what each has to do.

Numero Uno: Who's the Boss

As I mentioned before, in our society numero uno is the individual. As a physician, I'm told I should follow the individual's wishes to the exclusion of the wishes or needs of the family, society, myself, other caregivers, or God. Dollars also enter here in a sort of subsidized free-market way. We guarantee insurers a healthy profit while trying to limit governmental funding of health care. What I spend on this patient therefore has an impact on everyone else in his or her health plan. But we haven't gone quite so far as to say that the patient has a responsibility to protect the payer's profits. Not quite that far. Very close. Very, very, very close. But not quite. Not just yet.

It's important to recognize that there are wide religious and cultural differences in the interpretation of who's in charge. Communist and totalitarian cultures tend to consider individuals as possessions of the state, whether that means the total mass of society or one guy with many big guns. In that circumstance, the state decides.

When vegetative patients' cases make it to the U.S. Supreme Court, there's always much rumbling about a state interest in "preserving" life vis-à-vis the family's or patient's right to self-determination and privacy. The debates over euthanasia, physician-assisted suicide, and "informed demand for maximal care" hinge on two questions: Whom do health care providers serve—the individual, the family, the payer, or society? And what are the legal and ethical limits of our responsibility to provide comfort, even if death is the only comfort we can offer?

Some Asian and Native American families express the very clear view that the individual exists *only* as an element of the family or tribe and that either the assembled opinion of the family or that of a matriarch, patriarch, or other elder is the one that matters. In such views the individual's wishes are secondary to the good of the community or hold sway only after consideration by the family or elder.

The deeply religious frequently express the idea that they have to do everything, even procedures the patient doesn't want, because Jesus or God will decide when to call the sick person home. This idea is difficult for me because often I don't know whether I'm doing God's or the devil's work in that context. If Jehovah or Mohammed or Jesus is going to decide, why don't they just decide to keep this dear person alive without my machines?

And there is a rising movement in medicine to make decisions at an institutional or community level. This situation occurs to a certain extent when a community or a payer decides where to put the dollars—for example, a new MRI scanner, patient care, nurses' salaries, or profits for investors. Daniel Callahan suggested one approach to "rationing" health care dollars by asking, "Will $100,000 buy one more year of quality life?" It's the sort of consideration being used today to decide whether to fund mammograms for women under forty, or under thirty, or bone-marrow transplants for cancer patients. And as discussed in Chapter 7, the "futility" debate asks when health care providers' decisions may supersede the patient's wishes.

What about the great unseen decision-maker, the soul or the spirit? We've all seen patients make astonishing recoveries or fall apart before our eyes for reasons we can't explain. With some patients, everything I touch turns to mud. For others, every word I utter is like a golden raindrop. Many times I've seen a patient complete what he or she needed to do—the letter, the reunion, the embrace, the battle—and be dead in an hour. Perhaps the soul always decides, though the decision may be diametrically opposed to what our ego says we want.

We need to recognize that in many cultures, in many individuals, the decision rests somewhere other than where white Western culture presumes it should be. At such times we usually consider our patients indecisive or irrational, "difficult" or "uncooperative." And

I'm deadly sure that at those moments they feel exactly the same about us.

Others' Roles for Decision-Making Around the Last of Life

The Patient

The patient is generally the decision-maker and stands center stage. He can opt to assign decision-making functions to a surrogate, the family unit, the doctor, or a friend—many do. When that happens, there's much more than just a transfer of authority. Trust and responsibility are given in return for an unspoken promise of faithful nurturing. One requests that another's love, protection, and understanding be demonstrated. Near the end of a long life with many heavy loads to carry, you can just see the burden on a patient's shoulders become lighter when the weight of control is passed to someone dearly loved. "I want you to decide. See to it that I don't suffer if they can't get me better."

The Family

The family is seeing a tremendous history take a sharp bend in the road, perhaps to trail out of sight. The vast library of all the moments shared is about to close its doors. Whether we love or hate, fear or cherish our family members, they and the feelings between us have been there all the days of our lives. There's a cartoon titled "Final Last Tags" that shows a woman standing over a grave, looking down into it and declaring, "Did so!" Sometimes we hold on to this person's life as long as possible not only because we love her but because we can't imagine the world without her. "When Dad disappeared, Grandma took over everything—the farm, the family, what little money we had, all of our schooling and welfare. She was everything that held us together. Even though she'll never wake up, we'll fall apart if we don't have her here."

I don't know how *parents* survive losing a child, even a grown one. We bring our children into the world, see their struggles and victories, their wounds and healing. We invest a million hours of work, worry, and struggle and are rewarded with a delight that illuminates our very being. To go on in life without them must be like trying to walk with a wound as big as the world. In *Of Water and the Spirit* Malidoma Somé recounts his training as a Central African shaman. He says the *grandchild and the grandparent* are bonded because the infant has just come from the spirit world with news the grandparent desperately longs to know: soon the elder will be returning there. The parent is trapped in the world between, too far from the spirits to connect with them. To have brought your child from birth through infancy to adulthood and then to see your adult child revert through illness to dependency, helplessness, cries, and finally silence must be like standing frozen on a platform watching the night train barrel through and out of sight. In a time of such pain, parents may be forced back into earlier roles, making unimaginably difficult decisions.

Siblings often relive the bruises and adventures of childhood. The "hero" child who always took care of everyone and was responsible for their happiness, again has to shoulder their burdens and try to hold the ship together. The "difficult" sibling blows up at the hospital's cold inefficiencies and sneaks bottles of beer into the room. The scapegoat child shows up from somewhere back East and gets everybody so riled up that they forget how sick Mom is, today, in the brutally tense present tense. All the old wounds come out, yet we sometimes discover a fine rich note rising out of the cacophony. The deep strengths and commitments that have been misplaced along the way surface to coalesce the best of a family out of all the disparate parts.

Grandparents in tribal societies are often seen as those with the strongest connection to the spirit realm and hence best prepared to guide the sick person along the the path to death. In hospitals they've been replaced with social workers, head nurses, and a few senior doctors. How I long for those wondrous elders who knew how to take the helm through the darkest storms. Today our elders usually seem lost, adrift, horribly out of place in a world that has passed them by.

Friends

Friends are family by choice. Very often they've assumed the role of sister or brother, mother or father, or child. Odds are they can spend more time at the bedside than many family members can, and the odds are better than even that they know the patient's wishes, fears, goals, and hopes better than anyone else. Nurses are modern medicine's model of compassionate friendship and the ability to be truly present. When they're not consumed by endless streams of lab tests or buried beneath stacks of pointless documentation, nurses remind us all how to bring our deepest humanity to the work of dying.

Children

Children come in at least two varieties: young and grown. I'm not sure how much their actual age has to do with these categories. Perhaps it has more to do with how close they are to the spirit world from which they came, and what period of their childhood they're living out when suddenly faced with a parent's illness. One mother said to her forty-year-old son, "I just want things to be good between us, like they used to be." When he asked what time precisely she was referring to, she said, "When you were four." At the time, I thought this exchange was pretty weird. But now that I have my own young children, or they have me, I realize how precious these times are. And I realize that many of my patients' adult children are driven straight into a time warp: they become dependent or fearful, afraid of abandonment. They try to act grown-up, which they are, but they feel so powerless in the face of the illness that it's an act full of bluster and quick fixes. Part of them is in childhood, but part has become for the first time the strong parent to their own parents, now grown unsteady and childlike.

When my father had heart surgery, I became simultaneously a little boy tripping in a long white lab coat and a grown man, a physician, afraid I'd get caught letting my dad down once again. I was quaking inside and scared silly I'd get him killed and everyone would blame me and I'd be the bad guy again and my sister would be sure I meant to polish him off and my youngest brother would resurrect the time I bashed his nose with a baseball and threatened to bury him if he told our folks and it would just prove again that my other brother was right not to go into medicine. In the way that hero children do, part of me started getting irritated that here I was having to take care of everybody again, and who was taking care of me?

Then I remembered: this time I actually was grown-up, it was appropriate for me to be the caretaker, and no one was going to beat me up if Dad took a sharp left turn toward the nearest cloud bank. From that point onward, I managed to be an adult at least, oh, maybe 10 percent of the time, which wasn't bad, all things considered.

The exclusion of young children from the end-of-life experience in hospitals today is as grotesque as it is tragic for all participants. Over the years I've invited these little ones more and more readily into even the most horrific and terminal situations. Contrary to all expectations, they're intrigued rather than terrified by the tubes and gadgets. They bring an air of healthy, honest love, into medicine's black box. In every step, every breath, every flush of a cheek, they declare that life goes on. We're part of a continuum. Life heals even as it wounds; we are all that close to the spirit world.

Nowadays I talk with the entire extended family, with all the children and babies present, and discuss the clinical situation (also known as "the mess") from beginning to end. Constraints of time and differences in background limit our ability to cover everything. But every discussion should include the clinical situation, the outlook, who has what to decide, and the likely consequences of each possible decision. I let the children know what we're talking about, what the patient is experiencing, what they themselves will experience. I try to convey what it's okay for them to say or feel or do, which is everything and anything. And that it's okay if they want to come into the room, but it's also okay if they don't and just want to remember Grandpa the way he was the last time they played with him. Children almost always choose to come in, and I can feel their tension lift and everyone's healing begin the minute they come through the door and touch the pale hand lying there on the sheets.

The Health Care Team as "Community"

As death has been driven into the hospital, each of the nonfamily roles that cluster around the last of life has been reassigned to members of the hospital crew. These roles may shift, and the players may perform them in different ways, but it's good to keep them in mind and notice either when someone is playing that part or when you're putting them in that role for some reason of your own.

Among the job descriptions that come to mind I would include:

The Elder

Traditionally, elders carry the weight of experience and compassion for the members of the tribe. They hold this body of wisdom at the gate between this world and the "Other," the world that is invisible, beyond, after and before life. As the elderly have become devalued and isolated, this crucial position has been vacated in most situations.

The Judge

This role is usually assumed by the doctor, the administrator, the head nurse, the psychological consultant, or a hostile relative. Resented for his or her power, often cynical or controlling, the judge is a great one to blame. At the same time, it's reassuring that you can turn toward the judge for a firm answer, and by God you're going to get one.

The Patriarch

This is the role of spiritual conduit, usually assumed by the chaplain or the social worker. As a source of wisdom and connection with the ancestors, it might be taken on by an elder nurse or physician or a visitor from Hospice or the Cancer Society.

God

With the exception of cardiac surgeons and neurosurgeons, doctors have grown a bit wary of this role. The best we can muster is a priestly assortment of strange gowns and mysterious sanctuaries where we do things mortals aren't permitted to see. It gives surgeons a real head start on us internists. But to the extent that the power to heal or destroy is ascribed to us and our ministrations, rather than to the resources of the patient, we often are granted godlike powers by our patients. For the most part I think we use them well. Some of God's best moves were probably in giving Her children the challenge of free choice and the burden of knowledge: it's in these areas that today's would-be healers need a lot of work.

The Lodge

Many if not all tribal societies had lodges where members committed major parts of their lives to a common pursuit. There were warrior lodges, spirit lodges, healing lodges, and lodges for a multitude of other purposes. From what I read, each usually contained members of various ages, young and old, so the sacred signs and knowledge could be passed down in absolute secrecy. Revelation of such arcana to one not of the lodge could destroy the power of the medicine.

I think this notion captures the sense of ward units or work groups in the hospital better than any other model. We learn a vocabulary of five thousand words going through medical and nursing school and talk in a latinized shorthand that separates us from those not of the lodge. "Redress the fibular disarticulation t.i.d. with Ringer's three-quarter strength and Dakins." "Do you think those are PVCs or APBs with aberrancy?"

Power and magic are nourished by the assembled energies of the lodge. But isolation and the potential for abuse lurk there as well. Members may tend to confuse their views with truth. What made the lodge valuable was its absolute commitment to the good of the tribe and its unswerving adherence to the goals of the society. If you feel excluded from the processes of your health care team, you're dealing with a lodge gone bad, and you should demand access to the club.

The Minyan

In many traditions a group of ten men is necessary to convene a congregation of the faith. The minyan is like the leaders of the lodge, only without acolytes. In the hospital I suppose we convene our minyans in the doctors' lunchroom or the Nurse Practice Council. Administration boardrooms and the innumerable committees that devour our lunch hours and our spirits are just crawling with minyans.

The practice of making decisions about a patient's fate in secret back rooms has grave risks. How opaque or transparent is the process? Why should the patients and their families not see the uncertainties and power plays that determine their treatment? When and to what extent should families' and friends' input be sought? Angry families often sense some dark conspiracy. Why else does everybody come in one day demanding consents for more procedures, only to insist the next day that we should stop such aggressive measures? The minyan should meet in the open, and the family should participate whenever possible. It's been my experience that the more the various physicians and nurses involved in a patient's care interact in the presence of the family, the safer we all feel. Even our conflicts may serve to clarify those within the patient's immediate community.

The Witness

This is a role we seldom recognize but one that is perhaps the most crucial. The witness honors the person and the events by taking them in, being aware of their meanings, and testifying to history and the world about how this unique individual left the world. A compassionate witness can resolve the terrible isolation of a death or illness and help the survivors see the meaning of their suffering in the greater context of their loved one's life and society's desire to support them all through a hard time.

We who spend most of our working hours in hospitals are the familiars of death and disease. We can bear witness from a deep experience that gives perspective to the horror and weirdness of what's going on here. Yes, those stages of denial and anger, rage, bargaining, and depression are entirely appropriate. Here's what each phase offers. Here's what your spirit is calling for through these pains you're feeling. Here's where to stand, here's what you might want to do. Here's how to lean into the pain to feel more deeply the love of which it is a part.

We are so terribly busy *doing* in the hospital and at so many levels preoccupied with the *results* of our doing. The current vogue for evaluating doctors and hospitals is "outcome-based reporting." This approach attempts to boil everything down to quantifiable results: mortality, costs, length of stay, percentage of complications. The qualities most crucial at the end of life are those least amenable to quantification: compassion, empathy, patience, humility, appreciation, and the willingness to serve as witness to the passing of one precious being.

Goals for Each Participant

At the surface level, we presume the goals are pretty clear: patients are here to be cured of their illnesses. Families are here to support and protect their loved ones. The health care team is here to shoot down the illness with the clean, well-aimed bullets of medical technology.

As mentioned in Chapter 4, the questions addressed in considering end-of-life decisions should be much more about goals and the soul's purpose than about procedures. The illness should be a beacon, a shout, a warning. Listen very carefully to the plea within the disease. Listen very carefully to the plea within the "dis-ease"—the uneasiness, the world out of kilter that manifests itself in this illness. In this context, each participant on the stage has goals and needs far beyond the simple ones of beating the problem to death.

The *patient's* issues in addressing the Advance Directive, mentioned earlier, apply to all aspects of end-of-life decisions. We can apply the same list to everyone in the room:

- Goals
- Hopes
- Fears
- Quality of life before and after this illness or intervention
- Specifics of the clinical situation and its likely outcomes
- Burdens of therapy proposed
- Benefits of therapy proposed

Family Members

The family members' set plays out like this:

Goals: What do you hope your loved one can achieve through this illness? What old hurts, what unspoken loves or wounds, what unresolved issues need to be addressed now? An old woman, a survivor of the Nazi concentration camps, had lived out her life isolated from her family for forty years. By the time her daughter flew in, the mother was in coma and terminal. For the first time in all those years, her daughter held her hand and cried there beside her. She told of the deep appreciation she felt for the love her mother had tried to give. She told her about the qualities of her genes and spirit that lived on in her grandchildren. The old woman's tears ran too, and she became peaceful. I believe much was healed.

Hopes: What do you hope will be different after this illness or death? What would you like to do, or say, or be like that never quite happened before?

Fears: Of what outcome are you most afraid? In what ways are you fearful that you, or the hospital, the family, or society, may fail your loved one? What are your deepest fears about what your loved one will fail to be for you? What do you fear about life after the illness or death of your loved one?

Quality of life before and after this illness or intervention: The disruption in life's flow is a clarion call to ask what has been missing, what got misplaced, what has gotten stuck in the relationship of this person to the family. What happened to the love or joy? How did we forget to sit on the back porch and appreciate the sunset? What happened to quietly cherishing the other's presence? What happened to the letters that used to open the heart, or the touch that calmed the day's furies?

Specifics of the clinical situation and its likely outcomes: Suddenly faced with the possibility of losing your family member, what is this illness calling on you to find in yourself? The impact of the illness, and the likely outcome, are pertinent to all members of the family. Everyone will be affected by the experiences of the next few days and the new structure of the family after discharge or death. Every illness is really an illness of the entire family, and in many cases reflects the dis-eases, the wounded uneasiness of society as a whole. As I'll describe in Chapter 9, "When Society's Soul Speaks," it's likely that drug addicts, teen suicides, victims and perpetrators of inner-city violence, the family drunk, those whose hearts are destroyed by atherosclerosis and hypertension are just individuals carrying the burden of all of our shadow and pain. We can ask what this member of our family is carrying for all of us. What is her illness calling us to heal in ourselves?

Burdens of therapy proposed: Our society expects the caregivers, family, and friends around the patient to fulfill some Good Samaritan image or the role of the selfless servant. As embarrassing as it may be, I believe we need to be more honest about the burdens the therapy will impose on the family and caregivers. Family members should be permitted to consider how much they are being asked to give. How much of our life's other demands will have to be put aside to care for this person's problems? Where in my hierarchy of responsibilities does this illness fit? Which of my responsibilities is this illness calling me to reexamine?

In "amicus curae" briefs to various lawsuits, Catholic dioceses have addressed the question of our moral responsibility to sustain life at all costs. The general response was this: if (as individuals or supporting family members) prolonging another's life distracts us from more pressing competing demands (caring for our children, keeping our family alive financially, performing our responsibilities in our community), we have no moral responsibility to prolong life. If the burden of supporting that life is so onerous that it blocks us from feeling God's love and appreciating His bounty, the benefits do not outweigh the burden.

Families are often angry or offended when I suggest that their burdens, their pain and suffering, should be considered in deciding what to do about an illness. But for many patients, the impact their illnesses will have on their families is a very real part of the pain and fear they experience. A person may spend a lifetime building an identity, a family, a legacy. The choices he or she makes in the face of an illness may affirm and solidify this legacy or destroy it. We need to be much more honest in recognizing, honoring, and responding to the impact on the family.

Benefits of therapy proposed: The benefits of improving an illness or lessening a pain are clear and desirable. But if we can add to these the learning and healing within the family, we expand the power of the hospitalization immensely. What impact will the illness have on the days or years that will follow?

Health Care Providers

Health care providers are often trapped in a Florence Nightingale or Marcus Welby mystique that isolates us from our own humanity and limits our value by closing our eyes to what Carl Jung would call our own shadow.

Much of what has been said for the family applies to health care providers as well. We are, however, different in that when the patient leaves the hospital we don't carry his problems the rest of our lives, and because when this one leaves another one appears. Through all this we're expected to be clear, compassionate, caring yet rational. Many of us were hero children, many from dysfunctional or alcoholic homes where we were taught to care for everyone but ourselves. Like most hero children, we find that part of us seethes at this imbalance and is readily hurt when we discover ourselves treated as invisible or taken for granted. This dynamic gives a particular twist to our role on the stage of the last of life.

Goals: Our overt goal is the correction of the patient's illness. Our true goal is healing—healing our patient, the family, and ourselves. We came into health care for many reasons, but at least in part as an honoring or a corrective reenactment of what we learned to do as children: Through healing others, can we heal ourselves as well? Many of us are working toward unconscious questions awaiting answers— Can the truth be spoken at last after so much damaging silence? Is there a purpose to all the pain? Will I be able to fix in my patients what I couldn't fix in my family? What is my worth? Where is the joy?

Hopes: We hope that we leave at the end of the day feeling the world is a bit better for our part in it. That we reach across all the demanding busyness and conflicts to feel a human touch. That it not all be for nothing.

Fears: We fear that we'll fail again. That we won't be enough. That we'll be sued. That no one will ever notice how totally we put our hearts and souls into this work. Paradoxically, our cloak of professionalism often hides exactly that which we most want seen and acknowledged.

Quality of life before and after this illness or intervention: It's another patient, another bed change, another set of laboratory tests, and another terrified family. What can we learn or share this time? Why were we brought together in just this way? Why do the families and patients that most affect me feel so much like a part of myself I forgot along the way?

Specifics of the clinical situation and its likely outcome: Great anguish is associated with this issue in critical care around the end of life. There may be an immense difference between what the nurse feels at the bedside through a ten-hour shift and what the doctor experiences in a ten-minute visit. Labs and x-rays may not reveal the same information as the strain in an exhausted face or the dozen calls from a family in conflict.

The clinical situation is that many more illnesses are ameliorated than are cured. Thirty percent of patients admitted to the hospital will die. Death in the hospital is a miserable and wounding meatgrinder that traps us all. The prognosis is clear: we can fight death but are destined to lose. Even when the occasional battle seems to be won, we can welcome death as a wise colleague and be open to what this brush with death is willing to teach us.

Burdens of therapy proposed: Nurses are particularly loath to admit that part of the reason they feel life support should not be prolonged is because *they're* suffering—they feel like torturers; they feel that their energies and spirits are being squandered to no purpose or to an evil one; they go home at night drained by their grief for what they've done to this patient. We can deny such feelings, but they're fearsomely real. They show up in our family troubles and divorces, our wrecked lower backs and chronic pains. We pass them on to our kids and our friends as inevitably as we do our love and care. These feelings become part of the illness. The empathy we have with our patients and their families, the part of us that feels what it is like to be in the bed and around it watching someone who has grown dear to us undergoing horrifying changes, evokes our best qualities. By being honest about the burdens we feel, we offer our hearts as sounding boards to those for whom we care.

Benefits of therapy proposed: We have more experience with the limits and likely outcomes of therapies than do our patients or families. We owe them every bit of honesty we can give.

But there is a benefit we seldom acknowledge, which is how this illness and our response to it fulfills us. I want to include here the school assignment of Andrew Campbell, the eight-year-old son of one of our cardiovascular ICU nurses. He began by quoting a poem by Emily Dickinson:

> I heard a Fly buzz—when I died—
> The Stillness in the Room
> Was like the Stillness in the Air—
> Between the Heaves of Storm—
>
> The Eyes around—had wrung them dry—
> And Breaths were gathering firm
> For that last Onset—when the King
> Be witnessed—in the Room—
>
> I willed my Keepsakes—Signed away
> What portion of me be
> Assignable—and then it was
> There interposed a Fly—
>
> With Bule—uncertain stumbling Buzz—
> Between the light—and me—
> And then the Windows failed—and then
> I could not see to see—

I chose this poem because it is one of my mom's favorite poems and it means a lot to her. She is a nurse and has been with patients when they were dying.

In this poem a person is waiting to die. They expect to see god
and the last judgment but instead he just hears the buzzing of a fly
and then everything goes black.

What will things be like when we die? What will our last memory of earth be? My mom holds the hands of dying patients so their
last memory of earth will be a human touch.

In this short assignment, a young boy shows how far the ripples
of a patient's death travel and how much we can all be touched. His
mother's patients' deaths and how she attended them have been
passed to him, and through him will travel on to countless others.

Perhaps for each death we attend, we should all fill out Ken
Meese's form about dying well. What does the patient want, fear,
and hope for? What does the family look toward? What do we
health care providers need and hold as cherished goals? Were we
to compare our desires for the last of life, we'd be startled at how
much we share with the patients and families who seem so far removed from the workaday lives we only seem to live.

SIX

Into the Darkness: Discussing the End of Life

W E HAVE THE ISSUES and the forms, and now even the players on the stage. But what do we say? How shall we begin?

To speak well, we must first listen.

Communicating sensitively and effectively is always important, but never more so than when discussing end-of-life issues. Though the idea of listening seems simple, what we need to hear is often blocked by our fears, presumptions, busyness, projections, and flat-out naked terror. In these crucial moments, a quiet stillness may be far more productive than "doing something." We may be called on to receive the legacy or honor the uniqueness of the individual. Finally, we come face to face with our own rich humanity and its value, illumined by the way another human soul meets us in truth.

Caregivers and friends need to learn to be active listeners. We should listen openly, offering one another the sense of value that comes with having one's words truly heard and understood by an unguarded heart.

Our bodies speak and listen as well. By the way our eyes meet, our touch, the true expression of our emotions, we show that this person faced with death is still profoundly vital and present in our temporal world.

Even as the clock ticks and the waiting room fills, we must be patient. We're all too ready to finish another's sentence, conclude the incomplete thought, rather than face our own uncertainty. We need to take the time to parrot what we've heard, to turn it over in our own way to see if it still reflects what was said. Two decades ago, a white teacher wrote a book about the Lakota Sioux called *Hanta Yo*. She had it translated into Lakota, then back into English to be sure all concepts fit the Native American way of structuring thought and language. Between any two of us may lie even greater chances for misunderstandings and, by their resolution, learning.

In general, we should abandon "yes-or-no" questions; it's in the gray areas of "what-ifs" that one's values are truly revealed. Go more to the "why" or "how" of an issue than the "doing" that only pretends to be clear. What I mean will become evident in the dialogues that follow.

Perhaps most importantly, remember that the soul speaks more through body and scent, through slight movements and the feel of the air, than through words. If the eyes behind the sharp statements appear confused or guarded, trust the eyes and ask them to carry you where they yearn to go. If the hands are clenched or the chest collapsing, the decision spoken to "go for it" or "do whatever the doctors say" may not reflect the spirit's plan.

It is said that poetry lives in the spaces between words. Learn to be comfortable with silences. They are necessary "time-outs" for everyone in the room to process their feelings about what has been said. Sometimes the most important next question is … to sit still, or to embrace someone who is coming apart, just because it's what you feel like doing.

The following scripts are not meant to be definitive or exclusive. In a sense, they're not even authoritative since the whole idea of soul work is to find the inner authority our ego so often obscures. But I have several reasons for presenting them. I want to make them simple. I'd like to make it clear that end-of-life decisions can be addressed in all sorts of settings. And I hope to provide an outline around which your own explorations may begin.

If you're looking for a situation like the one you're in, you'll find each discussion headed by a description of the scenario in which it might be used. Age is mentioned here more as a measure of competence to decide the issues than as a determinant of the "right" answer.

Here is another of the stunning paradoxes the shadow offers us: these discussions of end-of-life decisions, considered so painful and so aggressively avoided by health care providers, are the door to some of the mysteries we've been wanting to get back to ever since we were children. It's the same land where all the magic stuff waits in fairy tales and other primal myths. It's a place very ancient and earthy, where nature once again shows itself to be cyclic and self-healing. It's where little men with deep wisdom lurk in dark places. Witches have ovens here in which childhood is leavened and baked into nourishing bread, even as death bows its head in retreat.

In *Care of the Soul*, Thomas Moore describes Saturn's remote and slightly too chilly sanctuaries as places where we could face our depressions. We go into such shadowed places to be healed and soothed, received by great, silent trees. Exactly at the point where we finally admit we're lost, we begin finding our way home.

The Basic Discussion

Certain elements of what I tell my patients and invite them to consider are common to all end-of-life discussions. They go something like this:

"Here are some forms you can use to consider end-of-life issues. These have to do with your wishes should you find yourself facing a serious illness, the quality of life you feel is worthwhile, and goals for your life.

"The 'Durable Power' designates a surrogate to represent your wishes if you become unable to speak for yourself. The 'Natural Death Act' only applies if you have a terminal condition or coma.

I prefer the 'Quality of Life' directives that focus more on what you value, are concerned about, or hope to achieve. Those should be the real focus of our decision when a serious illness occurs.

"You can fill these out now or at any time in the future. But it's good to think about such things and discuss them with your family and especially your surrogate, someone whom you'd want to speak for you if you become unable to speak for yourself. It's also good to encourage other friends or members of your family, both those who are ill and those who are well, to consider completing such Directives.

"Each of us should think about our wishes for the last of our lives when that time comes. I hope you'll use one or more of these forms and bring them back to me with your ideas and questions. When you've completed the forms, you should have a copy available at home, in my chart, in the hospital record, and with your family or surrogate.

"The Advance Directive chapter includes examples of forms that may help you describe your wishes. You can contact the organizations listed to obtain originals of these forms. Alternatively, you can type out your own version, but if you do so I urge you to consider the 'What Needs to be Considered' guidelines of Chapter 4."

Obstetricians, surgeons, pediatricians and oncologists, among others, often refuse to discuss Advance Directives, either because death is not probable or because it is so likely that such a discussion would frighten the patient. What do we do in particular situations?

Scenario I	Health: good
	Age: any
	Likelihood of Death: minimal
	Setting: office or hospital admission

"Though you're very healthy and there's nothing about your situation that makes me concerned about your outcome, every illness reminds us that we should think about "What if?" end-of-life issues. An Advance Directive both expresses your wishes and protects your family from the burden of making difficult decisions for you if you can't."

⟶ *Basic Discussion*

Scenario II   Health: guarded
Age: any
Likelihood of Death: significant
Setting: office or hospital admission

"Though you may do well through this illness [or hospitalization], we both realize there is a real possibility that we'll come to some very difficult decisions. Any change in health is a good reminder to think about such issues as your wishes for the last of life when that time comes."

⟶ *Basic Discussion*

Scenario III   Health: acute illness
Age: any
Likelihood of Death: significant
Setting: emergency room or office or hospital admission, preferably with the family present.

"You know you're acutely ill and we don't know which way things will go. I need to ask you some questions about 'what if' you become very seriously ill.

"The first is how you feel about your life before this illness. Is it satisfying? Do you feel okay about your current level of function? How much burden would you want me to put you through to achieve this same quality of life? Are there things you feel you need to do or complete in order to feel you've achieved what you've hoped to in your life?

"Second, what quality of life would be okay with you after this illness? I ask this so I can get a sense of what outcomes you would find worthwhile. What do you most fear and what do you need, to feel your life is worthwhile? What outcomes would you judge to be unacceptable?

"In terms of procedures, would you accept life support (mechanical ventilation, CPR, tube feedings, dialysis, ICU hospitalization) if necessary to save your life? If I felt the illness were irreversible, would you still want me to try these measures, or would you prefer that I focus on keeping you comfortable? What would you want me to do if I felt you would be left dependent or living in a nursing home?

"If we had to initiate life support, but after a period of time (days, for example) it appeared that we couldn't achieve that quality of life, would you want us to withdraw life support and instead focus on measures to keep you comfortable or if possible get you home?

"I'll see to it that we follow your wishes. When you get settled in, you might want to consider the 'Quality of Life Advance Directive' with your family, and fill it out or discuss it with me further."

⟶ *Basic Discussion*

Scenario IV   Health: any condition
                 Age: any
                 Likelihood of Death: any
                 Setting: patient has a "Do Everything" or
                 "DNR" Advance Directive

"I commend you for having filled out your Advance Directive. Have you discussed it with your doctors or your family? Do you know what it says? What did you hope for it to say? There are a couple of areas in which Advance Directives tend to be unclear."

"Do Everything": "The box you've checked indicates, 'Do everything, whatever my likely outcome.' In what situations would you not want this followed? How much weight do you

give to pain, cost, or burden to your family; your appearance; or your likelihood of recovery? What outcomes would you find unacceptable? If in my best estimate you were going to end up in one of those unacceptable situations, then would you want me to stop mechanical life support and provide comfort measures?" These would include control of pain and anxiety, optimizing your ability to function so you can achieve your goals, and helping to arrange your remaining time in the setting, and with friends and family you want to have present.

"DNR": "The box you've checked indicates, 'Do not prolong my life if I have a terminal illness, permanent unconsciousness, or if the burden outweighs the benefit.' What if you have a terminal illness through which you're doing well and enjoying life? What if the circumstance that arises appears reversible? What level of certainty would you want me to have before accepting that your unconsciousness will be permanent?

"Are you trying to indicate that you don't want aggressive measures *under any circumstance*, or that you don't want to be kept alive in a condition you would find unacceptable? These situations are very different, and you need to state what you feel about each one.

"We need to make sure that it is very clear to caregivers, family, and your surrogate what you mean by 'burden' and 'benefit.' Please consider using one of the 'Quality of Life Advance Directives' or 'Dying Well' to clarify your wishes and your values.

"Once I know what burdens would bother you the most, and what outcomes you would find acceptable, then I will have a better idea of whether to initiate life support or not, and when to withdraw it and go to comfort measures if I can't achieve an outcome you'd find worthwhile.

"I'd like you to have your family here when we review this so they know your wishes and you can all hear that I understand them."

———▶ *Basic Discussion*

Scenario V   Health: unable to express wishes
                   Age: any
                   Likelihood of Death: significant
                   Setting: Patient has no Advance Directive or
                       has an Advance Directive, but this is an
                       unanticipated situation in which the Direc-
                       tive seems inappropriate. A family member
                       or close friend is present.

"Your family member [or friend] is very severely ill and may
need to be placed on a ventilator, have CPR, or undergo other
aggressive measures. Has she ever discussed how she feels about
life support? If and when she said 'no,' or indicated this decision in her Advance Directive, what sort of situations was she
thinking of? Is the present quality of her life satisfying to her?
Has she ever indicated what quality of life she would not find
worthwhile?

"When she said 'yes' to life support, do you think she was
considering reversible problems or prolonged dependency on
such machinery? Would she want us to withdraw the machines
and go to comfort measures if we couldn't achieve the outcome
you tell me she would find worthwhile?

"Please understand that I'm not asking what you want, or
what medical interventions I should use. I have to make those
decisions, and I know you want the best for her. But your
knowledge of what she would have found beneficial or burdensome gives me direction as to whether I can achieve an
outcome she'd appreciate. Your feelings are very important to
me, and I want to be sure you see that we're following her
wishes. But I don't want you to feel you have to carry the burden of deciding whether she'll live or die. Her illness will decide that.

"Based on what you've told me, I feel the current situation
is not one she could have anticipated, and not what she was

considering when she indicated we should not resuscitate her. Her current health status is one she finds worthwhile, and this may well be a recoverable illness. Therefore, I think we should use life support and withdraw to comfort measures only if after a reasonable time it looks like we can't achieve the outcome you tell me she'd find worthwhile. [Or, Since the prognosis now is for an outcome you tell me she'd find unacceptable, and since she couldn't have anticipated this, I feel it would be wrong to 'do everything,' as she indicated in her Advance Directive.]

"Does that sound like what she would be telling me to do in this situation? If so, I'll take the responsibility of acting in compliance with her quality-of-life issues and her values, rather than the DNR [or 'do everything'] that is so unclear in this unforeseen circumstance.

"Here are a couple of 'Quality of Life' Advance Directives and one called 'Five Wishes,' which you might consider filling out as you believe she would answer. I think they provide a good structure for considering her wishes."

⟶ *Basic Discussion*

Scenario VI   Health: unable to express wishes
Age: any
Likelihood of Death: significant
Setting: Patient has no Advance Directive or a directive that seems contrary to appropriate measures in this unanticipated situation, and no one who knows him is present.

Our actions here are drawn from empathy, compassion, respect for who we imagine the individual to be, and an ethics of caring. The audience to whom our "scripts" are directed must be our own sense of moral responsibility for the well-being of this unknown individual.

The guidelines that apply are:

- If in doubt, pick life.
- If you initiate life support and later find out the patient would not have wanted it, or would not have found the likely outcome acceptable, withdraw immediately. Withdrawal of life support is not murder; rather, each additional breath from the ventilator or technologic prolongation of life is delaying a natural process of death that was for a time interrupted.
- The "Natural Death Act" in the face of terminal illness or permanent coma is binding and must be followed.
- If we act contrary to what we think would have been the patient's autonomous wishes in order to protect ourselves from a possible lawsuit, we violate our ethical responsibility to act in the patient's best interests.

⟶ *Basic Discussion*

Summary

We have ventured into uncertain territory, seeking cool wisdom and the waters of healing, yet here lurk the beasts of our individual and communal shadows and a hundred unanticipated forks in the road.

When conflicts arise, they may reveal the soul's deepest message. How shall we embrace and resolve the battles that will show us the way home?

SEVEN

Finding the Way Home:
Conflicts and Their Resolution

Who Am I? What Am I Doing Here?

As you can tell from the preceding chapters, the stage holds more players than just an isolated patient facing the end of his or her life. Each illness, each loss touches us in different ways. Each participant brings a dozen agendas to the proceedings.

Our conventional ethical responsibilities to the patient can be depicted simplistically as shown in Figure 7.1. The various roles I described in the previous chapters establish a web of rights, responsibilities, and hopes that looks much more like the scheme in Figure 7.2:

1—The family supports and cherishes the individual; the family is shaped by and inherits the legacy of how their loved one lived the last of life. This legacy includes not only knowing how the patient died but also the comfort that the patient's wishes, rights, and autonomy were honored.

2—The patient is supported by society, giving back to society the sum of his or her life experiences, wisdom, compassion, and courage. Increasingly, the question arises of the individual's responsibilities (behavioral, financial, contributory) to society.

3—Health care providers should support and guide the family. If we move the patient and family relationships into the central position currently held by technology, health care workers become participants invited into a very long story rich with emotion and possibilities for healing.

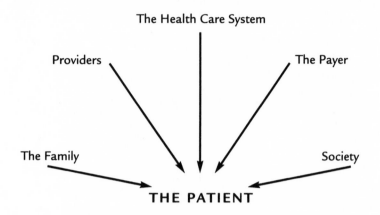

FIGURE 7.1 Our Conventional Ethical Responsibilities
to the Patient

The Health Care System

Providers

The Payer

The Family

Society

THE PATIENT

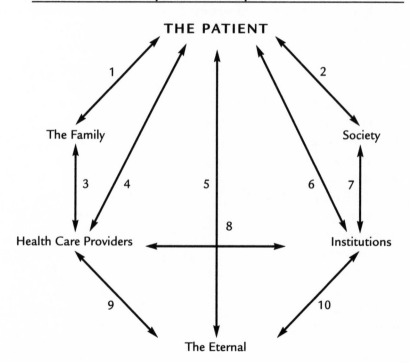

FIGURE 7.2 The More Realistic Web of Rights, Responsibilities,
and Hopes of all Participants

THE PATIENT

1

2

The Family

Society

3

4

5

6

7

8

Health Care Providers

Institutions

9

10

The Eternal

4—Providers offer patients skillful caring and give them grounds for hope. Yet the immense power patients have to touch and change those who care for them too often goes unnoticed.

5—Through death, the patient approaches the eternal while still living, from which viewpoint it is often possible to discover the meaning and justification for a life's struggles. The eternal, the ancestors, that which has been and will be imbue the illness with purpose. The thought of what will survive beyond death should affect what we each do and accept through the last of our life.

6—Institutions are expected to care for patients. But we are beginning to ask, What responsibility does the individual have to the institution? Must a patient undertake preventive care and cessation of harmful habits in order to "earn" costly interventions? If you smoke, do you lose your right to a ventilator? If you mistreat staff, can you be refused treatment? If you refuse recommended treatments, does the institution have the right to withhold other treatments made less effective or more costly by your refusal?

7—Whether by way of taxes, insurance payments, or legalization of such notions as preferred provider organizations (PPOs) and health maintenance organizations (HMOs), society funds and defines the means of delivering health care. "We, the People" determine what care is felt to be appropriate and provide courts to resolve disputes. The ethical principle of societal justice suggests that we have a responsibility to husband society's resources in a just fashion.

Our institutions have become the chambers in which those who comprise society experience the last of life—loss, grieving, transition, fulfillment, resolution, transcendence, or humiliation. By acting as the field upon which the last of our lives are acted out, institutions powerfully reflect back to society its values and how it views its members.

8—Health care providers and institutions are profoundly interdependent. Institutions provide the resources for us to apply our medical skills and have a substantial impact on the quality of our working lives. We in health care contribute to the reputation and survival of our institutions. We suffer and produce their traumas and in large part determine their viability. We fight tooth and nail for the health care dollar, much of which has slipped away to insurance company overhead and administrative costs before it gets anywhere near patient care.

9—Caregivers must redevelop a sense of the spiritual dimension of life. This gives meaning to what we do beyond the transient events of combating illness.

10—Institutions create the setting, the home, in which life is born into what follows this life. It is here that the eternal soul is touched, the legacy is given shape, the uniqueness of the individual is honored or tossed away. We are either reminded that we are all *one* or, in the confusion and rush, labor under the illusion that we are all separate. If we place ourselves in a framework where eternal souls manifest their needs and powers through illness and death, the hospital reestablishes its bond to the ancient lodge, the sanctuary, the Hospice. My office could begin to feel like a healer's hut somewhere in a mystic woods; the hospital bed around which the family mourns would take on the qualities of the altar in a smoky cave.

Conflicts

Conflicts within and between participants in the final drama are viewed not as windows on exactly what we came here to learn but as "problems," "aberrations," or "misunderstandings." A county medical seminar in San Mateo County in 1994 had the title, "Autonomy Versus Rational Decision-Making." I was a panelist in this seminar, with a lawyer and priest. At the time, I didn't quite catch the irony of the title. It revealed a number of assumptions that we take for granted:

- that patients and families are irrational
- that abstract rationality is the only "good" or "correct" way to make decisions

- that decision-making rather than witnessing is a health care provider's main function
- that such issues can be addressed effectively in a conference miles away from the bedside

Daniel Callahan wrote an article titled, "The End of Ethics Consultation," in which he suggests that hospitals should stop trying to resolve ethical conflicts in committees. Rather, he feels it's time to recognize that ethical conflict and resolution may be as common to illness as such physical details as temperature and blood pressure. It's likely that every illness brings up conflicts, a few of which reach the level of consciousness. Can we afford to pay for the treatment? Who is the decision-maker here? If the patient's lifestyle caused the illness, what are society's and the family's responsibility to invest money, emotion, and energy in the treatment? Who is responsible to whom for what?

More importantly, such painful places may hold exactly the key to the soul's search for meaning through the illness and impending death.

Conflict Resolution

Medical ethics is generally formulated around five or six essential principles. As understood today in America, most of these are focused on the individual, including:

Autonomy: This notion has been interpreted in such ways as "respect for the uniqueness of the individual" or "the right to refuse unwanted touching." The last few decades have added two other definitions that are really about power and fear rather than autonomy. These are "the right to demand and get whatever you want, no matter its efficacy or cost to the society or your ability to pay" and "why I (the doctor) have to do what the patient wants because otherwise I'll get sued."

Beneficence: The requirement that a physician's *intent* be to do good for his or her patient. For those who consider death evil, measures leading to a "good" death can never be beneficent. The intent to do good for the family, the community, our HMO employer, ourselves, or society is generally not included.

Nonmaleficence: We should not act with intent to do harm. The beneficence-maleficence equation is greatly affected by the weight we ascribe to several things, including death; low-yield, high-risk procedures; the moral, spiritual, emotional, and societal costs of suffering; and the impact on the patient and others of prolonged illness as a result of treating a particular illness.

Communication or Guidance: Informed consent, the cornerstone of our patients' right to accept or reject what we propose to do to them, is described as "adequately complete and accurate *bidirectional* communication." Chapter 6 offers some scripts designed to achieve such a dialog.

Societal Responsibility or Justice: This concept is a rough one. It covers such territory as deciding whether we should finance vaccinations for children or coronary bypasses for nonagenarians, preventive care or critical care, alternative health or ever higher-tech. This is the only component of medical ethics that doesn't focus on the individual patient. Societal justice is hard to apply at the bedside in the face of some of the gross injustices in how resources are made available in our society (see Chapter 9, "When Society's Soul Speaks").

Ethical conflicts over who is "right" and what "should be done" are resolved in several ways:

Denial: Most often, they're not noted to be conflicts, just uneasiness. The doctor goes ahead and writes her orders or the patient rails and refuses and is signed out against medical advice (AMA).

Bargaining: The conflicts are displaced onto scapegoats: if we can just wait until Tuesday, my husband will decide; I had a reaction to your medicine, so I don't want your surgery; we're upset because when our father died seven years ago, it took three hours to pronounce him dead; Mother's Advance Directive says she wants everything done, so you have to do it; if you won't stop drinking, you're not a candidate for a liver transplant.

The Sales Pitch: Many physicians have boasted (and I secretly agree) that we can convince a patient of almost anything. How we present the odds and the dangers, the outcomes, and the majesty of our intentions can sway most "consumers" to believe what we want them to believe. When patients don't fall for it, we label them "uncooperative," "a difficult family," "unrealistic," "depressed," or "demanding." In one recent ethics consultation, the surgeon was adamant that he hadn't "railroaded" the patient into accepting surgery. He had just informed her honestly that if he didn't operate, she'd die a "horrible, painful death." To the surgeon, it was futile not to operate because that choice would lead to an unbearable outcome. To the patient, an operation was futile because it wouldn't "cure" her problem. No amount of input from the other members of our committee was able to convince the physician that appropriate pain management and Hospice care would have provided a comfortable end to the patient's life.

Patients need access to a variety of clear, well-founded, sometimes contradictory information and guidance as to who is the decision-maker and what options are available.

Anger: Everybody gets pissed off and stomps out of the room (emotionally if not physically), and there are threats of lawsuits or abandonment. A risk manager materializes as if by divine intervention, trailing hospital managers and administrators oozing puddles of concern for the patient and family. But the person's title reveals their purpose: what is really needed is not a risk manager but an ombudsman, an advocate, a friend from within the system of care.

Nursing Intervention: Between the abyss of denial and the firefight of ethics consultation lies a mysterious island of humanity: the nurse who spends enough time with the patient and family to figure out what is really going on. It is from empathy and listening well that we resolve anguish into understanding.

A Family/Team Conference: Caregivers meet with the entire family to present all the information and the reasons for what we suggest. If it goes well, a few feathers get unruffled and people start talk-

ing. The nurses finally understand why we're writing such crazy orders and the doctors realize (perhaps) why our perfectly rational orders seem so crazy to the nurses. Somewhere in the muddle, agreement is reached, though this result is often understood differently
by each member of the council. "We'll try for seven more days."
"We'll do this but not that." "We'll reduce the pain meds so the patient can decide." "We'll get Hospice involved."

Ethics Committee Consultation: This is the penultimate minyan, the
lodge, sometimes the boys in the smoke-filled room. We assemble the
tribal elders, line up the judges without portfolio. Bereft of decision-
making power, fearful of liability if we document anything in the
chart, unsure what to write where, generally regarded by administration with a mixture of hope and fear, the Ethics Committee sifts
through the various interpretations of the data. What was said and
understood? What are the "moral bases" for the diverse opinions? At
emotional, moral, and spiritual levels, what is really the issue here?

Individual Rights Versus Futility: This concept captures the end-line
positions, the "two-minute drill," at this end of the millennium. Ac-
tivists for individual rights face off against Ethics Committee futility
guidelines. The Americans with Disabilities Act gut-punches the
Cost Containment Committee. Utilization review and risk management duke it out in the hallways, clipboards and monitoring forms
flying every which way. Everyone fancies him- or herself part of an
oppressed minority: the American Association of Retired Persons
(AARP) and the AIDS Coalition to Unleash Power (ACT UP) join advocates for the "other-abled." Nurses, doctors, and those with particular illnesses feel as slighted as do the medically indigent and the over-
burdened wealthy. *Nobody* feels they've gotten their piece of the pie.

Futility

I don't intend to slight anybody involved in these processes. As my
diagram suggests, we are all in a web of incredibly complex commitment, need, and sharing. But what I want to raise is the possi-

bility that *our arguments are at the wrong level.* I believe our efforts should not be about grabbing more resources, attention, or power. We need to shift from the battle for control to a deep search for understanding. The "futility" debate so heated in medical care just now is particularly illuminating.

Futility is a concept that has had increasing prominence in ethics literature over the past ten to twelve years. Lawrence Schneiderman, in dozens of articles and in books such as his powerfully written *Wrong Medicine* (with Nancy Jecker), has been particularly insistent and courageous. My sense is that futility is a child of the '80s, born of a desperate scramble to corral ballooning demands for infinite treatment. It's a response to the culture of litigation and our feeling of powerlessness—patients demanding everything for fear they'll get nothing; providers doing things they feel terrible about to protect themselves from the risk of lawsuits.

As described in the earlier case where the surgeon hoped to save his patient from a "horrible" death, the futility debate posits that if a procedure won't achieve its goals, it is futile. The hard nut at the center of this argument has to do with *who* will define the goals and *who* will decide the point at which those goals are so unlikely to be attained that the health care system needn't provide everything a patient demands.

As I write this, dozens of organizations around the country are writing "futility guidelines." Their purpose and questions are not entirely clear. In which situations can we refuse patients' demands for available procedures? In which cases can we do so without patients' consent or even their awareness? Who has the power to deem a procedure futile? On what basis?

Is a procedure futile only because it won't work at all or because it won't achieve healing, discharge from hospital, or a quality of posttreatment life the physician would consider worthwhile? Will futility be defined by those who pay for care, as in Oregon, or by those who need the care? When we finally admit that there is a finite pool of health care dollars, and that each dollar spent on me must be subtracted from the dollars available for you, which of us will yield?

Our discussions tend to be structured around such notions as what is "rational," "likely to succeed," "economically viable," or "not unduly burdensome." But this pretense of reasoned discourse leaves out the depth of emotion. Why exactly are we caregivers so wounded by our overdoing? Is it the money? Is it the waste of our own good hearts and efforts? Is it compassion or perhaps guilt for the pain our patients are asking us to inflict on them? Is it a sense of societal injustice? Is it rage that we're not really in control, that we feel our decisions are being made by CEOs and stock portfolio managers?

Or is it perhaps a raging hunger to return to what we really came here to do? Our deepest hope was to become healers of wounds, not the agents of perpetual wounding.

It's my distinct impression that most "futility" conflicts spring from:

- differences in goals, which we're reluctant to acknowledge or share
- differences in factual bases for our views
- the struggle for power in situations where we often feel powerless
- projecting our own judgments of ourselves onto others. This situation can be identified by using the Mirror Game, which I'll describe below.

If we're lucky, what comes of ethics consultation is a clarification of the first two issues—differences in goals and factual bases for disagreement. The last two, Third Chakra and the Mirror Game, are generally beyond the scope of "rational" discourse but in my experience are exactly where the healing waits to occur.

Goals: That which the daughter or the wife wants for the husband or father is not the same thing he wants for them and himself. What medical workers consider a successful outcome may be the worst disaster the patient could imagine. The nursing-home dependency we feel is an abject failure may be a very satisfying and productive outcome for the patient.

"This treatment is futile. It won't get her out of the hospital."

"Just having another two weeks to see my kids and hold their hands would be enough."

"I can't live without Mom. She's always been the mainstay of my life."

"She's three weeks past her DRG payment [which caps reimbursement to hospitals for her diagnosis-related group]. It's too costly to keep her alive in this condition."

"We must protect her from further suffering."

"She's a fighter. She'd want us to keep her alive in any condition possible."

"We're Christians. We must not abandon life."

"If my staying alive will help my children to come together again, then all of this misery is worthwhile."

Data: How often do we give the patients and families clear estimates as the basis of our recommendations? How often do we even dare to make a clear recommendation?

"With this surgery you'll be relieved of your pain, but you're perhaps 80 percent likely to die. If you survive, you'll have a 2 percent chance of being independent at home, the other 18 percent being various levels of dependency. Your average life span will be about six months. Without surgery, you'll certainly die. Here's what we could do instead to improve the quality of your remaining time."

"But we thought we had to do this surgery or you'd just stick Dad somewhere to die."

"Our uncle was on a ventilator for six months and has been well for years now. We could never forgive ourselves if we didn't try."

"Of 225 people with chronic lung disease who were on a ventilator more than three weeks, only two were alive at two years." That study's conclusion? "Therefore, it's worth trying for that survival by prolonged mechanical ventilation." How did the other 223 feel about their experience?

I've been impressed that beneath all the philosophy and compassion, the pleas and wise speeches, most ethics consultation crashes on the rocks of *control:* Who will get to decide?

Interestingly, the futility issue is the mirror image of the "right to die" and "right to refuse treatment" debates of the past two decades. Competent patients have won their autonomous right to refuse even appropriate and life-saving therapies. Now providers are struggling to regain the right to refuse treatments *we* deem to be insufficiently beneficial.

The Seven Chakras

Succeed. Benefit. Decide. How can we identify and grapple with the hidden energies and blockages that drive us? Eastern medicine and philosophy developed one view of our being a series of energy centers situated at various levels of the spine. The balances or blockages between these centers, termed "chakras," determine our health, our ability to respond to various situations, and our illnesses. In practice, we can feel the various chakras in action when our chest fills with love, our solar plexus tightens up in anger or dread, or we feel as if the bottom of our world is going to fall out when our survival is threatened. Our throat cries out to express our true will; our lower abdomen pulses with passion and sexual energy; we suddenly see clearly as if we had a third eye. Sometimes the top of our head tingles and seems to glow when we connect with an otherworldly, sacred energy.

As I participated in the range of conflicts that constitute ethics consultation, I became convinced that many if not most of the problems could be resolved by considering which chakras were involved. Similarly, the range of criteria various writers have suggested be used to judge a therapy futile can be examined from a chakra viewpoint—if one has enough backbone to do so (sorry—I couldn't pass up the play on words). Consider which level you go to when conflict arises.

The most important conflicts are those that involve serious or life-threatening illness.

Futility Chakras

Table 7.1 shows correlations between the futility discussion and the chakra system.

Our understanding and potential increase dramatically if we stop to sense at which chakra level we're working. It's my impression, strongly held and increasing daily, that most of our conflicts and even our attempts to resolve them are at the level of Third Chakra. In the midst of a heated ethics debate, we might look composed around the big wood table. But out of sight we're so tight, our guts would feel like an ad for "abs of steel." Disguised in civilized words and legalistic references, we're warriors struggling for power over this chaotic situation and over one another.

Who has the right to decide? When may we override the patient's or family's wishes? What does the hospital administration say we should do about this?

What are our liabilities if we write our opinions about the futility of continued therapy in the medical record? One article in the *Western Journal of Medicine* was titled, "What Does the Law Say?" Its point was that the law was a poor way to resolve ethical issues and that there are many times when we are ethically required to go against the law. A clear-cut example occurred in the county where I work. The Public Guardians' Office was refusing to permit physicians to write "DNR" orders for the office's elderly conservatees. In effect, these officials were requiring us to perform highly traumatic and ineffective resuscitations on the frail, demented elderly they were supposed to be protecting. Our ethical responsibilities to act with intent to do good (beneficence) and not to do harm (nonmaleficence) required us *not* to follow the legal mandate being imposed on us.

So what if we are working at Third Chakra? Who cares? I would suggest that everyone dissatisfied with how the last of life goes des-

TABLE 7.1 The Futility Discussion and the Chakra System

Futility	Chakras
The *futility* discussion ranges from "biologic futility" to "value to society."	The *chakra* system describes energy centers from the base of the spine to the crown of the skull. Like a xylophone, we play up and down these, but we and our energy tend to get stuck and never go any further.
Societal Value: Will the patient recover sufficiently to be productive?	**VII—Crown:** Spiritual, higher purpose, connection to the eternal and all that *is*
Societal Cost/Benefit: Will the intervention gain at least one year of quality life for perhaps $100,000?	**VI—Third Eye:** Vision, insight, understanding, clarity
Individual Cost/Benefit: Will the benefits of the intervention outweigh the burdens *as defined by the patient's value system?* Will the *patient's* goals be achieved?	**V—Neck:** Will, intent, focus, speaking your truth
Recovery: Is the intervention likely to improve the patient enough that she can leave acute care (or skilled nursing facility or intensive care)?	**IV—Heart:** Love, caring, connection
Fix: Will the intervention lead to resolution or cure of the specific problem involved at the moment?	**III—Solar Plexus:** Power, control
Improvement: Will the intervention cause measurable improvement even without cure?	**II—Generative:** Nurturing, creativity
Physiologic: Will the intervention keep air moving and blood circulating for even one more instant?	**I—Base:** Survival, connection to the earth

perately needs to care. First, our battles for power tell us just how much the illness is calling us to face the ways in which our struggle for control has harmed each of us—patients, family, health care providers. We're being told it's time to move from the fight into the heart.

Second, like some violent pile-up on the expressway, being stuck in Third Chakra blocks us from reaching the higher levels. If we believe we're debating Base Chakra issues of bare survival, or Second Chakra issues of death as the opposite of creation, we're confined to black-and-white absolutes. The point of this book is that illness and death call us to do the higher Chakra work that our hectic, distracted lives have so long helped us to ignore.

Third, being in Third Chakra traps us in the "us-them" dichotomy, reinforcing the separation and lack of communication that an illness urges us to transform into deep connection with one another. The appearance of power, like the flush of anger, disguises the powerlessness we all fear and keeps us from the interdependence that could offer true healing.

The Mirror Game is one good way to get out of Third Chakra. Envision yourself and someone who irritates you or who disagrees with you. You're sitting in two chairs facing each other. You begin telling the other what it is you can't stand about him. But as you begin speaking, imagine a mirror drawn between you. It's your face in the mirror. It's yourself you're actually talking about. The qualities that so enrage you or touch you, the views you find so repugnant, are just projections of your own image onto the other. This person is a mirror through whom you're finally beginning to know yourself.

Our preoccupation with power reflects our impotence in the face of illness and death. The power we envy in doctors or politicians, even the irascible patient, is our own power demanding to be honored. The addictions and violence that most repel us in our patients may be those we secretly yearn to experience.

When we accuse others of not loving enough, it's because our own love feels phony or puny. When we shout, "You don't see me at all," it's because we can't really face ourselves. Illness, death, and ethical conflict are some of the best mirrors ever invented. If we dare to look squarely into our own faces, they'll teach us just what we came to learn.

Higher-Chakra Ethics Consultation

Ethics consultation may be a discussion between a nurse and a bereaved, terrified daughter sitting at her mother's bedside. The formal versions occur in oak-paneled rooms where caregivers meet over greasy lasagna and sugary white cake as another lunch hour degenerates into turmoil and frustration. The tension may be between members of a family and the health care system or between an individual and the entire life she's lived. The discussion is usually formatted as "What should we do?" but I believe the real issues are "What did we all come here to this life, this illness, and this death to achieve?"

I would move the ethical debate as high up the chakras as possible, looking in the mirror each step of the way.

1. *Identify* who is disagreeing and get them all together. This group might include the patient, family, doctors, nurses, therapists, social workers, administrators, the bean-counter from the HMO, clergy, and lawyers.
2. *Communicate* the apparent disagreements and the current clinical situation. Be sure all concur that these are the areas of concern and that they've been depicted accurately.
3. *Elucidate* the basis of all interested parties' views. Crucial aspects include emotional, moral, factual, historical, ethnic, gender, motivational, and spiritual views.
4. *Identify* at which *chakra level* the conflict is occurring:

    Is it truly *Base Chakra,* about survival or death?

    Is it *Generative,* about a desire to give back to loved ones all they've given to the patient?

Is it *Third Chakra*? What type of control is sought? To what purpose?

Is it *Heart Chakra*? If so, everyone in the room deserves a rousing round of applause and a tremendous hug. They've escaped Third Chakra, gone beyond the fear and the resentment to the love we all came here to experience. Now, why is a roomful of love generating such divergent conclusions?

What is *Fifth Chakra, the Will*, the voice, trying to say? What is the patient's soul longing for us to hear? Does he need to show us what he's capable of doing? Is this illness manifesting the truth the entire family has had to keep quiet for so long? Is it speaking of a deep sadness, a remorse, an urgent need to forgive? Or is the will crying out that the time for forgiveness can't wait any longer?

What *Vision* is becoming tangible? What is yearning to be seen clearly at last? What does each of us really need to understand before this loved one passes away? Where are we being guided to go? What are we terrified to face, even though we know part of us will die if we don't?

We come to the *Seventh Chakra*, the connection to the *Spirit*, to higher purpose. Is this death and this process of dying in the hospital opening up our souls, or is it burying us deeper beneath even more of the rubble that's clogged up our entire lives? What can we do so our ministrations will open rather than close the access of this patient, all of us, to what is sacred?

I don't believe these ideas are all just mystical metaphor. The aspects of the soul that I enunciate in Part Five of this book, "Completing the Journey," all work and breathe at the bedside. When we touch on soul issues, the procedures become obvious. When we honor the meaning of what is happening, the outcome becomes less critical than how we approach the end that will be the next beginning.

When we escape the bondage of Third Chakra and surge into the next levels, the room changes. The abstract issue doesn't always get resolved; there's often no "rational" answer. But we begin talking from our hearts and from there everyone involved with this patient moves upward together.

One Patient's Journey Home

First Chakra—Base, "Physiologic." A seventy-eight-year-old woman on a ventilator and dialysis after eighty-three days in critical care says she wants to be kept alive. She's in pain, feverish, and malnourished with skin breakdown and open wounds. One son, desperately dependent on her financially and emotionally, demands that she be kept alive. The other son, who lives quite far away, is adamant that her suffering not be prolonged.

Second Chakra—Generative, "Improvement." The cardiac surgeon feels that the woman may survive and that dialysis is clearly prolonging her life. After all she's gone through, we want her to get some benefit from this brutal trial by fire. The patient feels her survival is necessary to draw her sons back together.

Third Chakra—Solar Plexus, "Fix." Another physician feels we can treat the patient's infection and perhaps get her to a subacute unit. There is open warfare between the two sons, the nurses, and various doctors about who should make the decision.

Fourth Chakra—Heart, "Recovery." There is no subacute unit that will provide both dialysis and mechanical ventilation, but the patient may be stabilized enough to go home, where she could die with Hospice care and her sons. She becomes tearful at this prospect and indicates that it would be a relief for her. Nurses demand that we acquiesce to her desires; the sons attack the health care team and each other over their disagreements. One can't live with the idea of her being gone; the other can't live with the idea of having failed to protect her.

Fifth Chakra—Neck, "Individual Cost/Benefit." The patient feels that if she can achieve the goal of getting her children to relate and back to Jesus, her life will have been sufficient. The nurses are devastated at the pain they have to put this defenseless old lady through, and at the conflicts between the sons that will prevent her last wish. Nobody feels their voices are being heard, or that their efforts are something in which they can take pride. What does any of this have to do with true healing? How does this circus honor the woman who is living the last of her time into dying?

Sixth Chakra—Third Eye, "Societal Value." The patient's care has cost $580,000. It's extremely unlikely that she'll survive, and if she does, it won't be for long. She has already exceeded one benchmark, $100,000 per year of quality life, by which we might judge the question of futility.

At this point, I would say the ethics consultation should focus on the vision she has for the rest of her life. The sons should be told what she imagines as her goal for them. If they are willing to attempt the rapprochement, and if her remaining alive a few more days will help them focus on that goal, then our interventions are not futile; her purpose is achievable and two other lives have their many years ahead to reap the fruits of their mother's vision. If the sons are not willing to pursue it, then we can't attain her goals for her, the scientific goals of returning her to health are out of the question, and we should terminate technologic interventions.

Seventh Chakra—Crown, "Productivity." This woman's suffering through illness has drawn the two sons into a tense but real physical proximity. It has focused us all on her values, burdens, and goals. We're all talking. She's experienced our love and our efforts to help her. I believe she's felt honored. With that ironic, compassionate chuckle described by spirits in near-death experiences, she's perhaps watched our drama with a growing understanding and some satisfaction. She may have found peace through this tortured process.

If the family and caregivers can open their hearts, their will, and their vision, their spirits too will be nourished by her last days.

"I know you want me to do this because you love your sister and don't want to lose her. But it's time for you to protect her from harm; prolonging her life may be the worst harm of all."

"It's breaking my heart that I'm asked to do these things to your father. And you're going to carry tremendous guilt about what we made him suffer. Let's see what we can do together to make the last of his life the best possible."

"I see your mother as a beautiful and brave woman who you tell me always cherished her independence and dreaded being a burden on her children. She was strong and held the family together. Now her illness has drawn you together again. What would she want you all to achieve, as a family, now that you're here?"

"If the grandkids want to come into the room, that's okay. Here's what you'll see, and this is what Grandma will be like. She can't talk to you, but she's not in pain. She'll know you're there. Your being with her will mean a great deal to her, but if you don't go in, she knows you're here anyway, and that makes her feel good too. If you want to hold her hand or kiss her, that's fine. It will help you re-member all the wonderful things you two have done together. And when her spirit leaves, you'll always have part of her with you."

"This is not about survival or death. This is not about fighting or giving up. This is not about caring or not caring. He'll always sur-vive for as long as each of you cherish his memory. What we're work-ing on together is building the memory he would want, and leaving him with the memories we'd want him to carry with him to what follows this life."

"What will things be like when we die? What will our last memory of earth be? My mom holds the hands of dying patients so their last memory of earth will be a human touch."

PART THREE

A Stone in the River

*T*oday I see that even death can be a form of
healing. When patients whose bodies are
tired and sore are at peace with themselves and
their loved ones, they can choose death as their
next treatment. They do not have pain because
there is no conflict in their lives. They are at peace
and comfortable. Often at that time they have a
"little miracle" and go on living for a while,
because there is so much peace that some healing
does occur. But when they die they are choosing
to leave their bodies because they can't use them
for loving anymore.

—Bernie Siegel,
Love, Medicine and Miracles

EIGHT

Technology, Slayer of the Soul: Our Struggle to Deny the Soul's Message

*H*ARD EXPERIENCE HAS forced me to the conclusion that the true tragedy of illness is not our impotence against death but our ignorance of how to cherish the value of a life. Our scientific focus on prolonging physical existence pays no attention to the unique purpose, learning, and healing that make each life, and each dis-ease, an invaluable gift. In the words of Norman Maclean, in *A River Runs Through It*, "It is those we live with and love and should know who elude us. The help we offer is not what is desired, and what is needed we cannot provide." In my line of work, our furious efforts to sustain the body may trample the soul that inhabits this body as the vehicle through which to achieve its potential.

Fear: Evading the Gifts Illness and Death Can Offer

The chapters of this section follow the painful journey we each will make from trying to evade an illness to the sad acceptance that we have no choice but to receive what the illness has to teach us. Our first response to discovering that stone in the river of life—that illness, the soul's mocking call, the threat of death—is to try with all our might to avoid it. Our first reflex is to plunge into the romance of *technology*.

It's important to understand that our technologic ability to affect the timing of death is only about fifty years old. Questions of which treatments to employ and whether or not to prolong life are evolving before our eyes. I believe that someday soon we will conclude that we've been asking the wrong questions all along. It's not the sums—the technology, the number of days or dollars—that matter. We should be asking the purpose: Where do we need to go? Which of the many possible routes will most likely get us there? What do we need to take with us, and what should we leave behind?

And why did each of you choose to join me on this mysterious journey?

When technology doesn't provide a quick fix, we fall back on *judgment:* What did I do to deserve this destruction? Why is my suffering justified? Why don't I deserve to elude my fate?

We bet everything on a *cure* as a way to escape the whole issue. But a cure may be the last thing we need: once cured, we can again deny the soul's call.

We arrange false dichotomies: Do everything or nothing. Live or die. Be healed (i.e., cured) or succumb. But at the end of life, it is the wound itself, not the cure, that reveals the path to healing.

When all else has failed, we *descend* into grief at our losses, our powerlessness, our knowing we have no choice but to face what lies ahead. That descent is in fact the beginning of the soul's journey toward the moment when we can grasp everything we came here to be. As will be discussed in Chapter 12, "Descent," grieving begins when we first have the notion that something may be about to change our life; facing the terror and sadness of this moment gives us the opportunity to explore our eventual death. By coming to terms with its lessons early in life, our death can inform us how we could choose to live the rest of our lives.

What awaits us if we move beyond the evasions, through the depression and grieving, into the work of the soul? After a time, squarely in the middle of all the terrible confusion, a calm descends on us and carries the pain into deep, still pools of comprehension. Viktor Frankl's "search for meaning" is engaged. It strides deliberately into the room and takes a seat beside its stalwart companion, Death. Steeped in profound silence and profound immobilization, a peace materializes that makes sense of everything that went before. The scent of decay yields to a suffusion of blossoms.

There were reasons for all the struggles. We rose above them.

They lifted us. They gave us all new life.

Our first step in this modern world is to travel through the twisting promises of scientific medicine in the following brief history of our relationship to illness and death.

Four Million Years: The Sounds of Silence (Acceptance)

Throughout this epoch, Death was accepted, ever present, and honored. The healer's role was that of priest and witness. There were certain "eternal" questions—how, when, where, and why to die— to which we will return after our fantastic fifty-year romance with technology.

Had I been writing this book even sixty years ago, the soul would have been considered a vital element in any illness or healing. For nearly all of humankind's history, as far as we can tell, any uneasiness of the body or the psyche, any dis-ease, was considered primarily an outward manifestation of spiritual problems. The gods were speaking, or the deep essence of the individual was crying out to be heard. A shaman was needed to enter a bizarre and life-threatening trance, to journey to where the spirit of the person suffering was doing battle with forces within or beyond itself that threatened irreparable harm. Through negotiation and altered perception, through sometimes life-threatening empathy, the healer grabbed the knowledge that was needed up above, on the surface.

During many thousands of years there was no physical technology to alter the designs of illness and death. We *accepted* fate and depended on faith to carry us wherever it could. Our healers were priests, rabbis, muftis, shamans, *cantadoras* and visionaries, saints and sacred stones. Our ills came from deep within us, or from others we had harmed. There was a blessing in every wound.

The few questions we could ask were almost childlike in their clarity:

Where will I die?
Who will be with me?
How will I be remembered?
What will live beyond me?
Who will speak for me when I cannot?

In times of epidemic or war, the fortunate or unfortunate few could add an extra question or two:

When will I die? (The warrior's cry, "Today is a good day to die!")
How? (Shall I flee death or face it? Will it be quick or prolonged? Will my last act be one of rage, or compassion? Will I prove wise, or prideful, or merely humiliated?)
To what purpose? (Will I die destroying others or protecting my own? What ends will my death serve?)

And always in the background or foreground loomed the hunger for eternity. In different periods, it might have been a hand outlined on the cave walls or a donor's portrait hidden in a church's stained-glass window. Some societies piled funereal treasures deep in pyramids. Others placed a bundle of cut flowers near a gravestone, resting in the cool shadow of cedars or oaks. All of them were questing after the answer to the question:

What does God (the Cosmos, Fate, my soul, my Master) hold in store for me?

We can find considerable reassurance in having a powerful, priestly presence to intercede between ourselves and the unimaginably powerful mysteries. But those same priestly figures have the potential to isolate us, to make us feel small and powerless. If they are unduly convinced of their power, they may try to ignore the reality that they are nothing more than one of us impotent little beings.

Then, abruptly, fifty years ago, everything changed as technology, the slayer of the soul, entered the picture.

How shall we understand the boundless faith and reliance on technology that have characterized the last half of the twentieth century? Elisabeth Kübler-Ross's path-breaking work, *On Death and Dying*, describes several stages in response to overwhelming change: denial, anger, bargaining, depression, and finally acceptance. Each of the last five decades of this century can be characterized as one of Kübler-Ross's stages. In each period we can discern a particular relationship between our humanity and our technology, between patients and caregivers, and between our notions of healing and cure.

Most of us facing end-of-life issues today have absorbed the lessons of these decades into our pores. Their patterns spring up in us today, often unnoticed or inexplicable yet powered by all the millennia of experience that preceded our own brief mortal time frame. Confronted with something so overwhelming as the last of a beloved life, we become one moment a child of the '50s hungering for an omnipotent, benign Father; the next moment we rock 'n' roll in the heady '60s hedonism of technology, only to become enraged adolescents of the '70s, demanding control in spite of our lack of information or experience. When the '80s scheme of bargaining with fate fails, we become depressed, immobilized, trying every '90s kind of trick we can to avoid what we see coming. Finally, we are forced to accept what we cannot maneuver our way out of.

Each decade of our tortuous romance with technology, each phase of Kübler-Ross's journey, contains much to cherish and much to discard. "To everything there is a season." If we can learn to recognize which period, which phase we're acting out of at the moment, we can draw from the best of that period what our soul needs to achieve its healing. And we can learn to resist the false promises and threats that accompany each way of seeing the world.

Some particular mode may seem familiar or troubling to you—
"Oh, yes, that's just how I feel." "That is how my doctor talks at
me—I don't understand how he could think that way." "I remember feeling, that's the kind of physician I would hope to be. Why
hasn't it turned out as I'd imagined?" "Is there any way out of this
feeling of hopelessness?" If so, try exploring the moods of that
decade. Each of the following sections offers some responses appropriate to finding yourself a patient, family member, friend, or caregiver stuck in the manner of a particular decade.

Nevertheless, two things are constant through this journey: soul
was put away in the chest of childhood toys that adult technology
no longer needed. And soul, demanding its voice, refused to rest.
What we deny in ourselves will be heard, even if in some dark and
twisted way. For each of these decades, I'd urge you to consider how
these views of the world are manifested in your current relationship
to illness and death. What about such a view impedes your movement into healing? What happened to soul in that decade, and how
can you bring your soul's purpose back into the light?

1940s–1950s: The Ascent and
Romance of Technology (Denial)

The nuclear bomb, polio vaccine, and iron lung led the wonders by
which technology claimed dominion over death. This was "denial"
of mortality based on a premise of military-style conquest. The
healer's role became that of patriarchal scientist.

In the half decade between 1947 and 1952, science snatched death
from the grasp of fate and faith. The atomic bombs over Hiroshima
and Nagasaki increased a thousandfold science's ability to make end-
of-life decisions for others. Iron lungs kept alive long rows of the victims of spinal poliomyelitis, and before we knew it Jonas Salk had
perfected a vaccine to prevent that tragic childhood disease.

America's industrial might and fancy machines had helped us win
the "Good War" in Asia and Europe. During the Cold War we came

to believe that our technology could conquer any enemy, be it the Soviet Union or Death itself.

By the early '50s, the shadow of those mushroom clouds and dark iron cylinders had driven the ancient priests into hiding. Laying aside their bone necklaces and gold-embroidered mantles, they donned the dark business suits of *Dr. Strangelove.* The old priesthood yielded to a new scientific, nuclear priesthood that derived its power from new abilities to prolong secular, physical life—or to obliterate all life on earth. The healer and destroyer, Shiva, had become fused in this new sect, which had no interest in the idea of soul.

Medicine followed the battlefront model of conventional warfare. On one side stood the doctor, backed with an armamentarium of medications and techniques. The heavy artillery of cobalt and surgery pounded away as new cures rushed toward the front lines. Across the smoldering field stood the disease, foreign and attacking from without. If the battle turned against us, we could call for reinforcements. By the end of the '50s, medical biology was well on its way to achieving the chemical and mechanical dissection of a particularly nifty, soulless machine called the human organism.

Many years later, I find myself asking, Where does the soul, that deepest essence that makes each of us human, stand in the battle? On a distant ridge, watching helplessly as the drama unfolds? Trampled beneath the rushing feet and the shifting lines? Blown away, nothing more than a wisp of acrid smoke? Did anyone care about such a question back in the '50s? Does anyone care now?

This pattern of belief lives on in our Intensive Care Units, where "everything must be done." One doctor commented, "When someone dies, we say 'We did everything possible.' We don't say, 'We put him through hell.'" When caregivers don't feel the need to obtain informed consent, or do so with almost no attention to the specifics of risk and benefit, we're living in the '50s. In the face of this cavalcade of whiz-bang technical stuff, such "soft" issues as patients' individual opinions or the desires of their souls don't seem terribly relevant.

The explosion of science achieved amazing advances and broadened horizons for the most desperately ill. But *who* our patient was, and the patient's role in the illness and its cure, slipped from view.

1960s: The Myth of Eternal Youth (Denial Continued)

The ascendancy of adolescence offered a new "denial" based on eternal youth, the sense of being a privileged group, and irresponsibility for the costs or consequences of our actions. The healer was now a relatively beneficent if remote father figure and provider.

Adolescence bursts with energy and fire, wildness and daring, intoxicating passions and the certain knowledge that the folks will foot the bill. With enough hormones and drugs, we would live forever. Sex, drugs, and rock 'n' roll would never die.

It was a confusing time for me as a medical student. Was I a kid living the great life our parents had won for us? Was I a victim of these cloistered power brokers threatening to send my butt to Vietnam? How had I become the bewildered "doc" treating overdoses and bad trips, raging alcoholics, and the sundry residues of too much great partying? The gap between patients and caregivers, between sons and fathers in the land where illness resides, widened. Patients had no idea what their doctors were up to but supposed they'd get whatever they needed. Caregivers had less and less an idea of what was going on under all those frizzy hairdos and beads but suspected it was nothing they were going to be happy about. And I, the son, was fast becoming one of "them," the fathers.

This chasm lives on today when we encounter a lack of understanding, verging on militant distrust, between caregivers and patients. For all our professed respect for patient autonomy—an individual's right to refuse unwanted interventions, or more anciently "respect for the uniqueness of the individual" (one definition of autonomy)—we caregivers know precious little about our patients, and they about us. Someone else still foots the bill—now it's our grand-children rather than our elders—and we generally expect someone else to take care of the problem. In denying responsibility for our own troubles, we gave away the belief that the power to address them resided within each of us. In the '60s healing power became something so foreign we barely knew it anymore.

We still need that exuberant, youthful optimism to make it through some of life's dark times. The fantastic otherworldliness of adolescence can provide a window into the life of the spirit. But we do have to learn that we ourselves will pay the price, one way or an-other, and that our fire and dreams, if not turned to the service of society, will wither and burn us down.

1970s: The Fall and Days of Rage (Anger)

Richard Nixon, Lyndon B. Johnson, Vietnam, and a growing aware-ness of science's perils moved us into anger. *Father Knows Best* be-came Darth Vader, the Dark Father. The first "right to die" cases hit the courts, and an idea called "Advance Directives" was developed to protect us from science's ravages when we became unable to speak for ourselves.

Something was dreadfully wrong. Death was romping all over the strawberry fields where we'd planned to play forever. By the end of the decade, fifty-eight thousand American youths would die in Asia. Jimi Hendrix and Janis Joplin couldn't imagine facing the '80s, and didn't. Two Kennedys and Martin Luther King Jr. were blown out of our lives. Everything seemed to be falling apart.

Someone must be to blame. Youth, parents, politicians, the CIA, J. Edgar Hoover, communists, blacks, whites, the poor, the wealthy. Suddenly we seriously doubted the good intentions, not to mention the competence or humanity, of those who had power over us.

In this climate community groups began drafting "Advance Di-rectives" as a peremptory strike against the ravages of technologic medicine. "Hell, no, I won't go" became "Hell, no, you won't do that to me." Little did they know how hard and confusing that battle would be.

I honestly believe that today's flood of malpractice suits and the resulting trend of "defensive" medicine are derived from rage at the failure of technology's promise of "better living through chemistry." False gods fall heavily, and often right on us. Distrust lurks between patients and doctors. We're hit with the implication that doctors are just in it for the money, that we keep people alive or let them die to suit our own purposes rather than theirs. Such views reflect the breakdown in trust between the recipients and the providers of care.

On the other side, those of us providing care are also enraged a fair bit of the time—at patients who harm themselves or don't participate in their care, at insurers that block payment or approvals, at institutions that don't provide the support we feel we need. Though rage feels empowering, it's usually misdirected, often at ourselves for being so powerless. It immobilizes us and those who would care about us. It burns away the silence, the sadness, the introspection that open the paths to our deepest yearnings.

Caregivers who feel attacked and mistrusted are unlikely to open their own souls to serve their own or their patients' healing. Patients who feel disenfranchised and powerless are unlikely to discover in themselves the resources necessary for their own enlightenment. There is indeed much to be angry about in how we treat each other in times of illness. Some of that anger will drive out the twisted foolishness so we can make our way back to the love.

1980s: Medicine, Inc. (Bargaining)

As business and the financial implications of medical care came to dominate medical decisions, bargaining superseded paternalism. Medicine introduced the concepts of "futility" and "resource management" to combat demands for infinite treatment. The healer became a gatekeeper, or a grocer offering treatments in unmarked brown bags. Increasingly, the timing and manner of death would be decided by committee, actuarial clerks, and CEOs.

In Washington a small army of accountants rose up and stabbed their No. 2 pencils deep into the eye of medicine. They invented a system of Medicare payment based on DRGs, or diagnosis-related groups. This meant averaging the cost of treating a given illness—say, gallbladder surgery—and fixing the amount of compensation to hospitals not at the actual cost of services but at a flat rate representing 95 percent of the going rate. If a hospital could do a procedure for less—get the new mom discharged four hours after delivery, do the gallbladder or mastectomy surgery as an outpatient procedure, not order the tests, not deal with other problems—the hospital stood to profit. If there were complications or a prolonged stay, the hospital lost big time. "Patients" had been turned into "DRGs," or that condescending term used by insurance companies and HMOs, "lives."

Suddenly, it was in our institutions' interests to do *less* rather than more, at least for Medicare patients. Our patients fractured into four tribes: Medicare recipients, who were pushed toward the least possible inpatient treatment; the privately insured, who mostly got everything; Medicaid clients, who got everything but for whom government paid at very low levels; and uninsured patients, who belonged at that other place down the street.

Physicians' practices began to fall under the baleful eye of the administrators and clerks where we worked. Some physicians became employees. From the insurance companies' viewpoint (and that of their stockholders), expenditures that actually went to health care, hospitalizations, doctors, and nurses were now termed "medical wastage." If I spent too much on patient care, I ran the risk of being dropped from the insurance company's provider panel. If my patients were too ill or had preexisting illnesses, if they developed costly problems or had too many needs, they risked becoming uninsured.

A great confusion prevailed in medicine: Whom were we here to serve? Were government, payers, and providers here to take care of the members of our society? Or was each of us here to serve the bottom line of government and the payer? Physicians had shriveled from priests to patriarchs to paternalistic bad guys—and now to grocers. Our long shelves were lined with brown bags marked "gallbladder surgery," "coronary bypass," "heart pills," "ventilator." Their contents were ill defined, their toxicities and health risks not described. We literally reveal more about a McDonald's burger than about the procedure about to be performed.

At the same time, our scientific and fiscal fascination with the quantifiable overpowered our recognition of the mysterious in who we are. Hospitals and providers came to be graded on whatever could be measured—mortality statistics, cost-benefit ratios, length of stay, number of lawsuits (whether valid or not), utilization of supplies and staff time. Forget how our patients and those caring for them felt, whether we healed and altered our lives or went right back to the same self-destructive habits. How did the illness change our views of the world and ourselves? These issues were not quantifiable and therefore didn't exist.

What was erased by all this bargaining and pencil-pushing was soul. There was no time for that "soft" stuff. Mobilize the patient's inner sources of healing? Who would pay us to do something like that? Spend time at the patient's bedside? Forget it—we had too much paperwork to fill out. For all the corporate mergers converting the community hospital into one tiny branch of Saint Megalopolis Health Care, Inc., the one merger that needed to happen became almost unthinkable. Healing comes from merging the spirits of patients, their families, and their caregivers into a circle of deep connection. There was no DRG for such an activity.

1990s: This Too Will Come to Pass (Depression)

HMOs, hospital closures, and medical indigence were the tip of the iceberg of our depression. The healer became immobilized, guarded, and uncertain. Advance Directives became widely available but were seldom used or followed. Studies confirmed the horror of death in America—prolonged, out of control, pointless, and ignorant of patients' wishes and values.

All the glorious achievements of medical technology in the '90s came crashing on the shoals of cruel financial schemes. HMOs, though started as early as the '50s, proliferated in the '90s like pin-striped bunnies. The hope was that they would do to physicians what DRGs did to hospitals. "Capitation" payments literally placed a price on the patient's head. Primary-care physicians would be paid for the number of patients in their practice rather than the services rendered. Even more prejudicial, physicians' incomes would be placed at risk for the resources committed to their patients. I could order a magnetic resonance imaging (MRI) scan or a coronary by-pass, but it would come out of my Physician Withhold Pool—that is, my pocket. Suddenly my patients became a threat to my own financial interests and those of the HMO that employed or contracted with me. Thirty to 40 percent of the health care dollar goes to the administration of insurance companies, billions of dollars go to lob-bying Congress against salvaging Social Security, yet we cut back nursing to bare bones so our hospitals' networks can turn a profit.

When we do get a procedure paid for, what do we really get? The technology that absorbs 15 percent of our gross domestic product can wound us in ways we never imagined. A patient can sue her payer in order to get a bone-marrow transplant for breast cancer, only to die of graft-versus-host disease from the transplant she finally receives. The brilliant new heart medicine encounters the over-the-counter antihistamine and causes a fatal heart rhythm.

The '90s question was not what my soul seeks or what healing I need; it was whether a clerk somewhere would approve the treatment or test my physician reluctantly ordered. Patients, families, and caregivers all felt powerless, hopeless, abused, constrained. This wasn't what we came here to do! What happened to caring? What happened to the meaning of Life and Death? Depression like the one that has seeped into so many health care providers' bones over the past decade means it's time for a change. Our soul has had its fill of not being heard. There's nowhere left to go but out of here. There's only one thing left we haven't tried: the authentic.

Yet it is in precisely such dark gardens of immobilization and help-lessness that the soul waits. Think of Luke Skywalker in *Star Wars* descending into the ancient forest. There he meets his dark father and slays him. Behind the shielded mask he discovers ... himself. Our patients, even our caregivers, are getting the first glimpses of themselves beneath the rubble. Some are turning toward visualiza-tion, inner exploration, hypnosis, healing touch, herbs, and spirit journeys for their own healing. Acupuncture is being touted as a valuable coparticipant in surgery and medical treatment. Cancer therapists are finding that group support, a search for that which is authentic in ourselves, and lifestyle change may be not only re-sponses to illness but in some cases the way to a cure. If caregivers would listen to ourselves, we might hear in our burnout, anger, and divorces the voices that tell us this path doesn't work. What became of your soul? How will you be a healer if you deny what is aching in yourself?

2000: The New Millennium (Acceptance and Beyond)

We have the opportunity to explore the eternal questions, now with the nuance of choice. We must look toward issues of meaning, pur-pose, and goals of the last of life. The healer will become the elder so vital to all societies.

After fifty years of the exhilaration of technology, we are coming back to ourselves and to the original questions. We can return to an informed, saddened, but more powerful version of Kübler-Ross's *ac-ceptance*, back where we left off fifty years ago. But like Inanna in the Sumerian myth I refer to in Chapter 12, no one returns from so powerful a journey unmarked. Our obsession with the false promise of eternal life has taken us to the outer reaches of our ability to con-trol life and death. Out there we discovered the consequences of denying our own souls. Having experienced each of Kübler-Ross's stages, our society is approaching the time not only to accept death's reality but to investigate the gifts it holds.

It is once again time to ask:

Where do I want to die?—In a hospital? At home?

Who do I want with me?—Who needs to share this part of my journey?

How do I want to be remembered?—What will be my legacy?

What do I want to have live beyond me?—What meaning, what purpose is my life intended to reveal?

In times of illness:

When will I die?—How much burden of therapy will I accept?

How will I die?—What quality of life would I find acceptable? If I can't achieve this, how will I craft the time I have left?

Faced with the joyous, bewildering burden of choice:

To what purpose do I wish to be kept alive?—What do I have left to complete?

Who will speak for me?—Who will be my surrogate? What of my wishes do they need to know? How will I communicate my values to them? What is it they are to say in my stead?

How in heaven's name will I ever find out what God has in store for me, if they won't let me out of this body?

NINE

When Society's Soul Speaks: Damning the Patient

To render the predator's energy and turn it into something
else can be understood in these ways: The predator's rage can
be rendered into a soul-fire for accomplishing a great task in
the world. The predator's craftiness can be used to inspect
and understand things from a distance. The predator's killing
nature can be used to kill off that which must properly die in
a woman's life, or what she must die to in her outer life,
these being different things at different times.

—Clarissa Pinkola Estés,
Women Who Run with the Wolves

THIS CHAPTER IS FOR the part of each of us that feels judged, unacceptable to our society or ourselves—disenfranchised, displaced, not good enough.

Society's soul, like that of each individual, reveals itself through its response to illness and death. That manifestation can take many forms, from sympathetic support to condemnation and abandonment. We are shown our meaning to society in part by how society sees or causes our illnesses. We determine how we see ourselves by how we respond to the environment around us in our most troubled times.

Most of us fall readily into the victim's posture—"they" made me smoke or work too hard or bathe in carcinogens or fall from the ladder or ride my skateboard into traffic or not get a mammogram. This approach is no less debilitating than society's tendency to blame the victim—she "deserved" to get AIDS or heart disease, that ulcer or cancer. It was a result of her bad habits, lousy morals, and general failure to behave herself.

In response, a New Ager may declare, "Ah, but we all create our own reality, so whatever misery befalls us we arranged." Across the table, a pious believer may contend that God is all powerful and therefore intended this illness for you, or even worse, that your illness constitutes just wages for your sins. I'm pretty hazy on just how different these two interpretations are. In our era of glorifying self-esteem, we soften the blow by contending that a beneficent God of Love must be laying this hassle on us for our own good and because we sure as the devil need it. Or we can congratulate our omnipotent selves that since we create our own reality, we've brilliantly devised all this misery for our own education. In either case, we know whom to *blame*. There is value in each view: the first urges moral rectitude and good behavior as a precautionary measure to avoid paying the penalty of illness; the latter encourages introspection, growth, and revelation rather than victimization. Each drives us in its way and offers us opportunities for spiritual exploration.

It's Them, Not Me

Almost every one except Mother Theresa maintains that blaming attribute, vibrantly alive and highly dysfunctional. I and other physicians are no exception. Since such thoughts are not politically correct, I keep them quiet even to myself, so I'm blinded to my own prejudices. But I will admit right here in print that I feel differently about those who harm themselves or others than I do about some lady who gets hit crossing the street. I'm severely short on sympathy for folks who try to dump all the responsibility for their care on others, then savage us for not fixing them up better.

And I do blame society for some of the nonsense I perpetrate. I recently sent a totally demented man to surgery that will prolong his life for years. Though they say he's been pretty at ease with his last ten nursing-home years, I can't get myself to feel good about the next ten that I (as society's instrument) just decided to inflict on him.

I don't smoke, so I smugly suggest that if you smoke and get lung disease as a consequence, you don't deserve time on a ventilator. But if you got your lung disease from doing construction work around asbestos, or from dust in the air, or from driving to work, then you've earned your ventilator. I love rich food, so I think coronary bypasses are excellent and well-deserved investments. I can't for the life of me get my brain to shut off enough to meditate, so the idea of requiring a course of meditation, stress reduction, and a 10 percent fat diet before considering surgery leaves me flat as a squashed lotus.

I think these judgmental and damning attitudes are the cruddy runoff from the battlefront mentality that slices our world into dichotomies. "They" deserve to die for their moral bankruptcy or greed, bad habits or rotten position in the scheme of history. "We" deserve to live for our upstanding decency, technologic wit, and obvious blessedness. One study of ethnic attitudes in medical ethics went to such an exotic place as Iowa to discover that the good folks there felt that race and nationality were not valid criteria for providing or withholding medical resources. Anyone who had worked deserved equal medical care. What was missing was the fact that nationality and race may have a great deal to do with a person's ability to get work, to perform it without encumbrance, to become "legal," and to make enough money to buy insurance.

Us and them. I and this damned disease that's come upon me. The fix that will cure me and make me whole. The healer and the healed. We use these right-or-wrong judgments to keep ourselves from looking deeply into the eyes of others who seem at first so unlike ourselves. But in those eyes we will ultimately discover our own true reflection. In what follows, I will use two illnesses that particularly capture the "them-or-us" dichotomy: AIDS and coronary heart disease.

He Brought It on Himself (Blame)

A character in the movie *Red Sun Rising* says, "In America, when there's a problem, we want to find out who's wrong. The Japanese want to find out what's wrong and fix it." While I suspect that this particular dichotomy is as foolish as most others, the idea does reflect how comforting it is to find someone to blame.

But when the consequence is to blame an illness on the individual grappling with it, it's clear that the purpose is to isolate and judge that individual, thereby insulating ourselves from our own vulnerability. A remarkable number of homophobic politicians turn out to have gay siblings or children, and Congress has produced quite a number of "family values" advocates who turn out to have abandoned their families without anything resembling regret.

The list of scientifically demonstrable contributors to coronary heart disease includes cholesterol, high blood pressure, cigarettes, genetics, stress, personality type, salt, infectious agents (including one interestingly involved in a form of venereal disease), aging, gender (male), and lack of fiber. This list leaves out all the most deep-rooted factors we have acknowledged in poems and idiom for millennia: it breaks my heart; what a heartache; I left my heart in San Francisco; he hasn't the heart for it; her heart just gave out; what a pain you are; what a heartless deed; and what one radio station suggested as a title for an age-appropriate Rolling Stones song, "I Can't Get No Circulation."

We have a lot of positive or negative judgments about these contributors to heart disease. Americans have a deep ambivalence about wealth: we resent the wealthy though we hunger to be among them. Hence, "rich" food perhaps carries its own just deserts. Hypertension: a very nervous inner-city patient once told me she developed high blood pressure because "those people at work just make me so hypertense."

Cigarettes: if you're really putting it out there, you're "smoking" or "on fire." If you see a character lighting up in a movie, he's either a slimebag or more likely working hard, grabbing a moment's respite. Better yet, he's either working up to or recovering from some great sex. Genetic predisposition is the modern equivalent of God's condemnation, or the sins of the father being visited on the son. We have strong judgments about personality type: a hard-driving, rigid, overworked person is described as Type A while that slouch who's laid-back and easygoing is merely a Type B (or Brand X). Salt: For thousands of years a man has been defined as "worth his salt." Many of my Hispanic and Chinese patients have refused to restrict their salt intake because it will keep them from being "full-blooded" and virile. Infections: We haven't figured out how to blame people with bad coronaries for getting chlamydia, but the personality traits that contribute to heart disease probably infect those around the sufferer. The best we can do is blame folks with heart disease for getting old. The elderly, who used to be a tribe's most precious repository of memory and wisdom, are now seen as a drag on the system.

Fiber: We look with disdain on someone who doesn't "have the fiber" to tough out life. The gender factor is interesting: depending on your generation, sex, and nationality, maleness may be considered a very good or a very bad characteristic. But in general the qualities that characterize male behavior are associated with all the risk factors for heart disease. It's a manly sort of thing to keep your feelings in, lock your heart down, tighten that tie around your throat. A real man doesn't mind having crushing substernal chest pain and wouldn't even notice if his heart were broken.

AIDS is in many ways the other end of the spectrum. Whoever invented this thing was sinister enough to pick for its victims several identifiable, heavily stigmatized subgroups: gay males; intravenous (IV) drug abusers; prostitutes and their customers; prisoners; dark-skinned folks in the Caribbean, Africa, and Asia; hemophiliacs who become infected through transfusions of HIV-contaminated clotting factors and who carry the same genetic defect as the last czar of Russia; and women who have sexual relations with men from the other groups. Sex, drugs, and foreigners. Between Christian attitudes about the body in general and sexuality in particular and our elder generations' misgivings about everything from the '60s on to current popular music, it would be hard to find an easier bunch to condemn.

But then, what about children who acquire AIDS from vertical transmission at birth? Original sin! Or those who got it from a blood transfusion during cardiac bypass? Oops. Or the high school kids who do what high school kids have done since way before there were high schools but because they're white and suburban and studying hard don't think they need protection? What about when it's my brother, or my daughter?

The AIDS virus has had the additional malevolence to attack young, vigorous people who have no business being seriously ill. They don't look ill, at least in the early stages. They haven't worked long enough to deserve serious health problems. With the exception of health workers who get stuck with needles, they didn't become ill in the course of gainful employment. The activities that transmitted the disease didn't threaten the sales of any commercial enterprise of the scope of RJ Reynolds, American Brands, the American Dairy Association, the California Egg Advisory, or employers who like to see their workers just working their little booties to death.

Greek and other mythologies abound with stories of gods who ate their own young—Zeus, the Titans, the old men who send young men to war. Like the Christian God, Abraham was willing to sacrifice his only begotten son. So many ancient worldviews included infanticide that it must indicate something in us calling out to be heard. Our judgments about AIDS are part of a long tradition in which aging Saturn brings down fleet, hermaphroditic Mercury. One of the mantras of our elders about the transgressions of '60s and '70s youth has been, "You people all figure, if it feels good, do it!" For the

young, vigorous, sexual, or intoxicated to come up with a fatal disease may seem thoroughly justified to Zeus or the Titans.

Societal blame is a way to compartmentalize, to isolate the illness
and the ill person from ourselves. It's a way to justify neglect. It's a
way to convince ourselves that we're not susceptible because by being unlike "them," we won't get it. That's probably quite true: we
won't get it at all.

We become particularly schizophrenic when we approve of the
behaviors that led to an illness. A man who doubles over from a life
of hard work, who has become wealthy by carrying the load, acting
like a man, and toughing it out, has earned respect for his illness. In
fact, the illness proves how hard he lived. It's the coup de grâce, the
"hero" medal in the lapel. I've taken care of elderly Asian men who
developed renal failure because of urinary obstruction from a big
prostate. The requisite hours of squeezing to produce a driblet of
urine were one sure sign of aging. In these men's culture, unlike ours,
age brought great honor, a presumption of wisdom and status. Here
we get our prostates whipped out at the earliest sign of resistance lest
the young guy in the next stall laugh at the old geezer straining to
get it started. When I was stationed in Germany years ago, an elderly woman's status could be defined in part by the number of medications she laid out on the table before each meal. This one was for
blood pressure from so much anguish caused by her children. This
one for the ulcer from not eating regularly because she was too har-
ried. That one for the joint pain from all the loads she hauled. The
new one (hurriedly ordered when Frieda next door got another pre-
scription from her doctor) was for the rash from the harsh detergents
she wouldn't invest the cash to get gloves to protect her hands from
because her husband's car needed a new seat cover.

Illness has meaning. The treatments have meaning. But if we give
the wrong meaning, if we misinterpret the signs, we're left with only
a handful of blame and judgment, or on the other extreme false
pride, without compassion or revelation.

The question needs to go from "Who's wrong?" well past "What's wrong?" to "What's right?"

He Doesn't Deserve the Resources (Retribution)

Beyond isolating ourselves from our fears about being vulnerable to a certain illness or debility, blame permits us to withhold resources from "people like them." Consider the fears I described earlier about finding oneself on the "slippery slope." Americans have decided we must blind ourselves, pretending everyone has the same right to infinite health care, no matter what the likelihood is that such care will benefit the individual or society, or first thing you know, we—you—she—I?—will discover ourselves up a creek without health insurance.

This is indeed a politically and emotionally charged area, and one in which *why* we decide and *how* we decide tells us much more about our own souls and that of society than *what* we decide.

The Oregon Basic Health Services Act took the bold and long-needed step of admitting that the "pot" of dollars available for medical care was finite. Proponents of the act picked an amount of money that the public was willing to invest in Medicaid, then listed treatments from those most worthy of coverage (vaccination of children, cancer treatment and prevention, etc.) down to those least worthy (cosmetic surgery, for example). They started at the top and worked their way down until they ran out of dollars partway down the list.

The problem was that it was non-Medicaid folks who could afford health insurance deciding what care those on Medicaid would receive. And therefore those not on Medicaid could receive care unavailable to those on Medicaid. It was a brave, bold, and honest expression of what we've always known: our financial worth is linked to our "rights." Paradoxically, the most underserved group in America is the working poor who don't qualify for Medicaid but can't afford insurance. For them, nothing is available. The act tried to address that problem by providing care to all people below the poverty line. But the trade-off was to limit what type of care would be available.

Our federal government funds a vast military complex, $700 million helium depots for dirigibles that will never exist, and coronary bypasses for ninety-year-olds so demented they don't know they're alive. Yet it frequently refuses to pay for vaccinations for children. A soul statement is being made by our society. It's Zeus and the Titans again. As a dollar investment—in terms of how many years of healthy life we buy—vaccination, nutrition, and sanitation beat coronary bypasses by a thousand to one. An elder's life is as rich in knowledge, experience, suffering, and uniqueness as a child's is in potential, innocence, and hope. Both feel pain and fear, and both are deeply vulnerable. One has "earned" health care by a lifetime of effort, whereas the skill and commitment with which we nurture the young will determine the future of our society. The two lives are "equal" in value to the individual and their "right" to health care.

The devil is in the details. And the devil—the demon—the daemon or genius that is the manifestation of our soul—speaks in the complex, ambivalent contradictions of the details. What constitutes "quality life"? If being gay or dark-skinned or female is considered not as valuable as being otherwise, then that year of life is not worth as much.

Quantitatively, a life saved at eighty-six buys fewer years than one saved at two. In a society that too often considers both the elderly and children a burden, we're not at all clear whom we really care to save. Is that old man just a drain on society, taking up space in a nursing home as he gabs away his days, or is he a precious repository of a life's experiences and the wisdom that our society so desperately needs to relearn? Nursing homes and retirement communities are both a consequence and a cause of our sense that the elderly are used up, useless, without anything to offer. We don't see them because they're stashed away. We don't think they have anything to offer because we never think to ask.

For my part, I'll admit I'm imbued with a cultural view that gives great weight to consciousness. We have defined brain death as death. Every other organ can be going along swimmingly—the heart just teeming with emotions, the spleen coddling the soul, the liver swelling with life force, the lungs inspiring and expiring one breath at a time. The kidneys percolate along, filtering out criticism and shame; the fingers and toes still touch the sheets. All are doing dandy. But this person is dead.

So, given my judgment, I hate sustaining someone who is never going to "wake up." I feel even worse about caring for someone who is awake but so demented or crazy that her life seems like some zombie hell. Yet, remarkably, my medical career has moved inexorably into sustaining exactly such patients. What is my soul trying to tell me? Why does it make the choices that put me in such a place? Is it asking my mind to consider the possibility that mind is not all? Is it telling me to listen to what my own organs would speak if my big brain would just clam up and listen?

The Muffled Cry

As a nephrologist, I know a patient's lifeline is his IV access, usually a woven Dacron tube implanted under the skin. When this spot gets infected, the tube has to be removed by a horrendous filleting of the skin, at the staggering cost of a prolonged hospitalization and multiple other attempts to get access to the circulation. I had several patients in San Francisco who kept infecting their grafts by shooting up drugs, and each time it enraged me. I desperately wanted to say, "The next time, no more. We leave it in and you die." There's really no legal or ethical way to insist on such a thing. But mustn't there be some point at which a person's choice to harm himself absolves society of the responsibility to save him from his behavior? Is it compassion for our less fortunate brethren or the realization that we're cowering in our glass houses that keeps us from defining such a point? There's no question that I blame and judge; the question is whether I can learn what these feelings tell me about myself and my purpose in working with such patients.

If we move from "what to do" to the level of soul, we're nudged to ask *why* a patient did what he did, and why I resented it so. What was he crying out? Was it that he wanted to die? That the only highs in his life were the drugs, that his life was a slum burning down in the fever? Was it only in the hospital that he could feel the master of other slaves? For a few days did he relish having power over us, if over nothing else in his world? Did he hate himself so much that he was going to make himself pay?

And was my rage the intellectual disapproval that he was wasting all the money, time, and effort we were investing in him? Or was it something deeper? The idea that IV drug abusers don't deserve to live? That they're accessing a pleasure I don't dare take? I remember a T-shirt from the '60s that declared, "Reality is for people not strong enough to take drugs." Did I find it intolerable that he popped drugs that made him feel high while all I took was the call, night after night, for me to put him back together again when he finished partying?

I heard his judgment of me! Was he saying that my care for him was worthless? My disgust was revealing a hidden part of me—what I would describe in Chapter 12 as my Ereshkigal—displaced, unacceptable, unvalued. If I truly admitted how it felt for him to devour my days and nights, I would have to acknowledge that the message I heard was this: "You may give your life, your health, your freedom, and your happiness to serve me. But they don't mean a thing. Your efforts will never be enough. You didn't try hard enough; you didn't do the one thing that mattered; so you're of no value. I cast you aside like the fool you are."

We were two souls deeply wrapped in historical wounds and projected translations, screaming at each other in a room that was to all appearances silent. For all I know he's still shooting up today, devouring resources by the bucketful, and his physicians are still making a good living off him and hating it.

As Larry Dossey points out in *Meaning and Medicine*, there is no illness without meaning. To see no meaning in the illness is an illness in itself, perhaps the core illness of medicine in modern times. There is no choice free of value judgments. We cannot "ration" resources, no matter how "rationally," without manifesting a value judgment about who "deserves" a resource, how much they "earn" the care or "lose" their rights by contributing to their illness. When I place myself in the position of judge, I declare my values proper and my debilities nonexistent.

But what we can do is try to become more honest with ourselves. Why do I keep a man alive in coma on the ventilator at huge expense? Is it because I don't know what constitutes a life worth living? Am I afraid I may end up sliding down somebody else's slippery slope? Does my soul know that a person is much more than a mind and that the soul lives on in my brother? Or is it just because my institution and I are willing to roll up a profit at great cost of suffering and delusion to the patient, his family, society, and those who demand such a farce? As with all of the soul's contradictions, the answer is "Yes." All of these issues motivate me. Some are calling me to know what matters most in me. Some are calling me to release the deceptions and errors my ego has imposed on the true path of my life in this world.

I have no doubt that treatments for AIDS were delayed because the disease was showing up in minority groups that were not highly valued by the political powers that be. It's very likely that the terrifying and tragic explosion of AIDS in the Third World is being facilitated by the First World's (how's that terminology for a judgment?) views of what people of color and people who have unprotected or homosexual sex deserve.

And I have no doubt that Zeus and the Titans are munching away on their children when we vote down bond issues for schools or refuse to pay for vaccinations for our children. Our soul is speaking in these choices, but it's the soul of a society showing itself so deformed, so self-destructive, that one day we'll leave ourselves no choice but to listen to our collectively and individually ignored souls.

This Is My Cross to Bear
(Guilt, Shame, Denial, Rage, Bargaining)

Perhaps even worse than societal blame and the consequent with-holding of resources is how we do the same things to ourselves. When I have a tooth pulled, I expect complete anesthesia—laughing gas and a comfortable chair bobbing on a sea of Muzak. And I get it. When a woman has an abortion, she's run in and out of a clinic so fast there's no time for sedation or adequate analgesia. The scream-ing is added, layer upon layer, to the two emotional screams from deep within. Why do we treat these two extractions so differently, and what shame makes the women in the latter case accept it?

I'm a doctor, and therefore I run on a motor fueled with guilt and shame. I know I've done *something* wrong; I know that every per-sonal-injury lawyer in the country knows it; but I'm just not sure yet what it is. My medical school professors and clinical proctors assured me I'd never be perfect like them, and every day I prove them right. Therefore I go to ridiculous lengths trying for perfection. I remem-ber every failure or mistake and forget the thousand tiny acts per-formed well.

The real mystery for me in this area of self-blame is those who don't feel shamed and culpable for their problems. I've never seen a smoker decide, well, I got myself into this mess, and surely no one else has to bail me out with a ventilator. I drink and eat too much but surely won't decline my bypass when the time comes. We set up incredibly stressful lives, turn away from quiet and contemplation, then wonder why "they" haven't made the pill that will help with this depressing anxiety.

Yet beneath all of this blissful hedonism lies knot upon knot of self-blame. I sense that each of Kübler-Ross's stages is in part a strug-gle with the issue of self-blame and responsibility. Let's say I am discovered to have a medical problem. I *deny* the illness because it is something awful within me demanding to be heard. I am *angry* at the illness and the messenger because they threaten the precarious agglomeration I've built to keep myself together. I *bargain*, hoping to distract myself from the message, hoping not to have to face this fact about myself. I become *depressed* that I have no alternative but to see myself as ill. But depression also takes us to Saturn's isolated garden grove, that narrowing passageway where change becomes inescapable. In Saturn's cold, distant realm time stands still while something dark bubbles and brews with icy determination. My eyes turn inward; nothing will be permitted to move until I at last see myself truly and well.

Then I realize how much I arranged to reveal this particular disease within me, how I delayed responding to it, blamed myself for my pains, and therefore carried them too long. I became identified with the illness and refused to give it up. And because I felt I deserved these pains, I created more and more of them. If I feel unworthy of love, I precipitate blowups with those I love because their love feels false to me. If I hate working, I become a workaholic to punish myself for hating it. If I seethe with resentments and rage at my powerlessness, I turn these judgments on myself—my stomach that eats itself away, my heart, my cells that become cancers, my tissues that turn arthritic and inflamed.

Finally I arrive at Kübler-Ross's phase of acceptance, which I think we usually see as acceptance of our illness. But as I write this book I realize how much this phase is really about acceptance of ourselves—the story of our lives—and our soul's message. Oh, so that's the music my soul wants me to hear. Oh, so that's what I'm about. I see now how much I condemned myself, arranged the rejections, precipitated the crises, felt I deserved to be sick. I've come here to understand why I imposed this punishment on myself.

As we move from self-blame and condemnation to embracing our wounds and needs, we can learn from the ways in which we accepted society's burden. We have wounded ourselves and others so often in

our quest for power. When we release that struggle, we finally discover our true strength. I blame myself, condemn myself, create my
own illnesses and diseases, and then berate myself for having them.

I and my soul are powerful enough to demand a voice. Illness is
one way we can speak. The God who brings the illness is the God
who can cure it. The virus that kills, slightly altered, becomes the
vaccine that stems the epidemic. Even blame is a light by which I
and my society can show ourselves exactly what we need to heal.

TEN

The Illusion of Cure: Hoping to Escape

*Does this not bring to mind the story of Death in
Teheran? A rich and mighty Persian once walked in his
garden with one of his servants. The servant cried that
he had just encountered Death, who had threatened
him. He begged his master to give him his fastest horse
so that he could make haste and flee to Teheran, which
he could reach that same evening. The master consented
and the servant galloped off on the horse. On returning
to his house the master himself met Death, and
questioned him, "Why did you terrify and threaten my
servant?" "I did not threaten him; I only showed surprise
in still finding him here when I planned to meet him
tonight in Teheran," said Death.*

—Viktor Frankl, *Man's Search for Meaning*

If I Can Just Get Rid of this Illness, I'll Be Okay (Illness as Separate from Self)

The illusion of a cure is perhaps the most unfortunate fairy tale we strive to live. Fairy tales carry information about the soul's needs and healing, about the stages of initiation by which we grow and transform, and about society's failings and hopes. They form the framework on which we construct our world.

My kind of medicine is built around a fairy tale that runs something like this:

It is a lovely and sunny kingdom (my body). Things are run by the old king and his three sons. (Oops—change is coming. The female element is missing.) But then a plague comes over the land (loss, deficiency). Invaders from far away descend, and there comes a great devastation (illness attacks from without).

The first two vainglorious sons (let's call them Learned Fool and Self-Righteous) go to do battle and are slain (wrong doctor, adverse drug reaction). The youngest son (that good-looking guy on the latest doctor show, perhaps) demands the opportunity to try his luck. Reluctantly, the old king sees him off (the right doc, the one who has a less staid or old-tradition view, the newest antibiotic just off the shelf).

Along the way, the youngest son encounters a little old man at the roadside (the clerk who decides treatment authorization requests at the HMO). Unlike his elder brothers, this son listens to this little man's outlandish advice (he knows how to work the system).

He proceeds through a series of trials (chemotherapy, spinal taps, dialysis, more adverse drug reactions). He is aided in his quest by magicians dispensing arcane wisdom (decked out in magicians' garb of surgical costumes as they merrily cut and sew). He frees the princess (the immune system), and they ride forth and drive off the invaders (cure the cancer or the infection). They return home to a triumphal procession (blood coursing through the newly implanted coronaries), and the kingdom springs into bloom (we all go off and play tennis, our golf bags filled with Metamucil, Viagra, and Grecian Formula 2000, our incontinence pads so petite they're barely noticeable).

The fairy tale we live in modern medicine is a simple one about defeating an enemy called illness. However, the real point of fairy tales, and all of life's deeper stories, is transformation, initiation, and unearthing the meanings that are at the core of our lives. The third son's job wasn't to find a bride. It was to bring the kingdom—our lives—back into balance. The goal of the "healing arts" is not to repel an illness but to discover what is wrong within.

Talk to someone a year after they've had coronary surgery. Odds are, their habits are nearly identical to those that contributed to the coronary disease. When death knocked at the door, it may have beckoned them to a quest: examine your life, attempt a rapprochement with your children, forgive your spouse and yourself. Prepare a legacy. Consider what follows life.

Most likely, that all stopped cold the day of discharge.

Omigod, a Cure: Now What Am I Going to Do?

Many AIDS patients described a profound confusion, even terror and outrage, when a group of drugs called protease inhibitors appeared. They'd already gone through all the stages of grieving to an acceptance that death was inevitable and imminent. They'd lived their lives and exhausted their finances, planning to be dead soon. Having walked through the fire to achieve an inner peace and calm acceptance, they had turned toward more spiritual tasks. Suddenly these new drugs promised a return to health and indefinite prolongation of life. *How dare you tell me I'm not going to die! What do you expect me to do now?* This reaction wasn't petulance or ingratitude. It was that ripping feeling of being pulled back from halfway to the other side, as ghastly a notion as being pulled back into the womb when you're halfway out.

Stephen Levine suggests in *A Year to Live* that we should all live one year of our lives as if it will be our last. If illness is one way the soul can get our attention, the cure is often the way we bludgeon the soul back into unconsciousness. Mel Gibson, stretched from a rope in the film *Maverick*, looks heavenward and barters: "Lord, whatever I did to piss you off, if you just get me out of this I promise to rectify the situation." We all look to God or the pharmacy or the government to save us. But how often do we make good on our half of the promise?

By Focusing on the Cure,
We Struggle to Escape the Learning

Were we to turn our time and strength to completing our earthly tasks, we might unearth the gift of healing transformation. In *Care of the Soul*, Thomas Moore emphasizes this point: "A major difference between care and cure is that cure implies the end of trouble. If you are cured, you don't have to worry about whatever was bothering you any longer. But care has a sense of ongoing attention. There is no end. Conflicts may never be fully resolved. Your character will never change radically, although it may go through some interesting transformations." A substantial part of our genetic material is viral, bacterial, reptilian, porcine, redundant, mysterious, and, in general, inexplicable. We carry it all, and perhaps every bit of it is meaningful to our being. We may indeed be much more the sum of the things that eat at us than of the things we eat. Our illnesses are like that too, recording in our wounds and how we respond to them the essence of what we prove ourselves to be. We can escape our illnesses only by escaping ourselves. If we look deeply into our illnesses for what they've come to teach us, we discover the chance to become whole.

Most tales of transformation begin with a descent. Whether we look to ancient myths of gods and goddesses, tales of ordeals and abuse, or the diary of a hospitalization, we begin with loss and end by being different than the sheltered being who began the journey. In this chapter I touch on only the first phase: the loss of our outer-world pretensions. We hold to these with the desperation of those who believe not that we wear them for a brief season but that they are our very essence.

Viktor Frankl described what seemed most important as he was brought into his first Nazi prison camp:

> I tried to take one of the old prisoners into my confidence. Approaching him furtively, I pointed to the roll of paper in the inner pocket of my coat and said, "Look, this is the manuscript of a scientific book. I know what you will say, that I should be grateful to escape

with my life, that that should be all I can expect of fate. But I cannot help myself. I must keep this manuscript at all costs; it contains my life's work. Do you understand that?"

Yes, he was beginning to understand. A grin spread slowly over his face, first piteous, then more amused, mocking, insulting, until he bellowed one word at me in answer to my question, a word that was ever present in the vocabulary of the camp inmates: "Shit!" At that moment I saw the plain truth and did what marked the culminating point of the first phase of my psychological reaction: I struck out my whole former life.

Jean Shinoda Bolen in *Close to the Bone* drew the parallel between entering a hospital and entering the underworld or a prison:

- One must pass a series of gates: the door to the hospital, the admissions desk.
- At each one, something is taken away: at the hospital room, for instance, street clothes which declare our individuality and status are replaced with a standard hospital gown that often is ill-fitting, too short, and flailing open up the back.
- In increments, thereafter, a patient is stripped of dignity, choice, and authority. He is transported on a gurney or in a wheelchair to radiology, the lab, or to have various scopes inserted into orifices. The gates into surgery threaten loss of consciousness or body parts, beyond which other gates lead into recovery or critical care.
- Psychological defenses are stripped away: denial, intellectualization and rationalization, addictions that keep feelings buried, activities, responsibilities.

Again, from Viktor Frankl:

Thus the illusions some of us still held were destroyed one by one, and then, quite unexpectedly, most of us were overcome by a grim sense of humor. We knew that we had nothing to lose except our so ridiculously naked lives. When the showers started to run, we all tried very hard to make fun, both about ourselves and about each other. After all, real water did flow from the sprays!

Apart from that strange kind of humor, another sensation seized us: curiosity.

When we focus on a "cure," the noise of our activity drowns out the silence necessary for the soul to do its work. We are busy hammering and twisting a stainless-steel bridge across the deep, tortuous valley of descent through which the illness would take us. Such hard times, such powerful callings cannot be evaded by technologic hubris. They demand silence and descent, humor and curiosity. A dark, mysterious valley stretches beneath each of us. It is too wide to span. We must descend into it and pass—haltingly, fearfully, but at last barefoot, very close to the ground—through it to ascend the other side.

ELEVEN

Shall We Do Everything ... or Nothing?

Paula came to my room again last night. I heard her enter with her light step and the striking grace that was hers before the ravages of her illness; in her nightgown and slippers, she climbed onto my bed and sat at my feet and talked to me in the voice she used to exchange confidences. "Listen, Mama, wake up. I don't want you to think you're dreaming. I've come to ask for your help ... I want to die and I can't. I see a radiant path before me, but I can't take that first step, something is holding me. ... You, Mama, who are always talking about your friendly spirits, ask them what my mission is, what I have to do."

—Isabel Allende, *Paula*

"SHALL I DO EVERYTHING, or let you die?" "Would you want us to do everything to save you, or not?" In a world built on yes-or-no answers and black-or-white alternatives, such questions are how we "give" patients a choice: life versus death. Care versus abandonment. The balance we offer is depicted in Figure 11.1.

How Did It Become So?

There are several bases for such an unbalanced proposition. I would include among them:

- The quantifiable: length of life, survival or death, billable procedures, and the "risk/benefit ratio" of interventions fit the scientific model of recognizing only that which can be measured, counted, and "proven." It is much more difficult to assign discrete values to the process of death, the afterlife, or the quality of the last of a life as a patient and the survivors learn the lessons they came here to explore.
- Secular belief that the soul and what comes after life is nothing: therefore, care that impacts the soul or the consciousness that survives death is by definition meaningless.
- Silence: since we've forgotten how to talk about death, we can't address our needs as we approach the end of life.
- Fear: when patients, families, or physicians prepare for death, we're accused of abandoning our commitment to life. We fear we'll "take away the hope." We're afraid of the powerless, out-of-control, dark depression that we will travel through in the next chapter. Just as we feel the abyss that yawns between what is known and what lies ahead, we feel that in an emptiness so vast, all effort must be pointlessly trivial.
- Isolation: few of us in this technologic world have experienced an intimate, communal healing process of dying. In too many instances, the family at the familiar bedside or around the home parlor, the rituals that honor and release the departing spirit have been forgotten. The ancient rites of grieving and reparation get trampled beneath the rushing feet of daily life. Never having experienced them, we believe they do not exist.

Or Should We Do ... Nothing?

At a recent symposium for Hospice volunteers from California and Oregon, I raised the question of this "emptiness," this "nothing" that we describe as the alternative to technologic heroics. What, I asked, can we place in this empty box? The answers flow from three

FIGURE 11.1 How We "Give" Patients a Choice

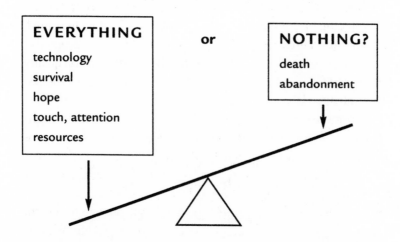

main questions: (1) What would you consider the qualities of a good or a bad death? (2) What do you hope to create for the dying patients with whom you choose to spend your time? (3) What do you come here to achieve for yourself?

Their contributions were:

- love
- peacemaker
- openness
- reminiscence
- guides
- empowerment
- sense of "home"
- be in the present
- understanding
- how to say good-bye
- letting go
- honesty
- compassion

- acceptance
- prayer
- listening
- sharing feelings
- touch
- hugging
- manicure (!)
- permission
- teach the rest of us about life and living

If we envision these and whatever other aspects of a "good" or "healing" last-of-life you might conceive, the balance shifts. Now it looks like Figure 11.2.

I would ask you to take one step further. Having seen that the alternative to "everything" for the patient is a "nothing" that in fact holds most of life's desires, take one more look. Those of us not yet dying who come to accompany death can fill the end of a life with the qualities these volunteers described. But ask yourself, what do we come here to receive for ourselves? Why did our souls choose for us to be present as this dear one's death approaches?

One wizened grandmother cupped her two hands and said, "I always touch the people I work with. Touch is very important. The hands are what they need." Looking into her eyes and that beautiful open cup, something in me cried out, "Darling, I wish I were dying. You could hold me forever." And I believe she'd have been willing to do just that.

FIGURE 11.2 The Alternative

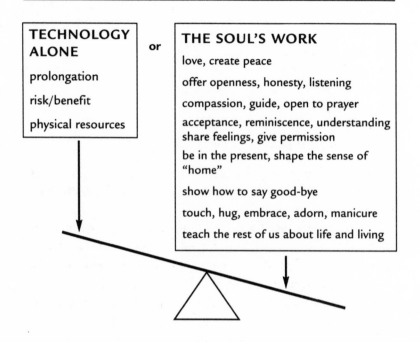

TECHNOLOGY ALONE

prolongation

risk/benefit

physical resources

or

THE SOUL'S WORK

love, create peace

offer openness, honesty, listening

compassion, guide, open to prayer

acceptance, reminiscence, understanding share feelings, give permission

be in the present, shape the sense of "home"

show how to say good-bye

touch, hug, embrace, adorn, manicure

teach the rest of us about life and living

TWELVE

The Descent:
By the Road of Tears Will
We Find Our Way to Healing

*I need to talk about my thoughts and fears. I am going through so
many changes; I feel so uncertain about my future. Sometimes all I
can see in front of me are those future things I am afraid of. And
each day, my fear ignites a different emotion. Some days I can't take
it in and I need to believe it isn't happening. So there might be days
or even weeks that I will feel sad, or act irritated. If you can listen
and accept me, without trying to change or fix my mood, I will eventually get over it and be able to relax, and perhaps even laugh with
you again.*

—Christine Longaker, *Facing Death and Finding Hope*

Who am I? What am I doing here?

—Ret. Adm. James Stockdale,
Vice-Presidential Debate, October 14, 1992

When the denial of the illness and denial of the soul have
both run their course, where do we go? When we realize
that technology will save us from having to face deeper questions,
how shall we act? What fearsome catastrophe awaits us in that black
hole of not doing "everything"?

We have so little idea of what to expect of illness and death that we fill that emptiness with all of our worst dreads. We feel isolated, helpless, abandoned. Totally adrift, we feel we are leaving behind everything we had hoped would save us in this life.

I want to take the time in this chapter to recount several writers' descriptions of "the descent." These are different journeys, on different subjects and from different eras, but the point I want to make is that they are all the same journey. Over thousands of years, at different stages in our lives, in times of loss or panic or dying, we all make the same journey over and over. We grieve the loss of a job, a pet, a loved one, a phase of life. A possession we thought we couldn't live without slips away or is never attained. Many things small and large escape us until, at some point, we face the loss of our own health, our own life.

My purpose in recounting these tales is not to depress you but to present depression as one necessary and healthy step we all must take on the road to healing. Nor do I want to frighten you, for fear is what so traps us in our present pain that we don't dare begin the soul's work.

Stages of Grieving

We fear grieving because it feels like a helpless slide into the abyss of depression. Yet it is exactly there, in that dark, lost place, that our soul will prepare us to return to our outer lives, forever marked by our experiences. One of the most painful aspects of this journey is the profound sense of isolation—I'm so terribly alone; no one can understand what I'm suffering; no one else has ever felt this hopeless. Yet the commonality of this passage can be sensed in the tales of countless writers. Figure 12.1 shows that as we traverse this valley, we can compare the terms used by Elizabeth Kübler-Ross in *On Death and Dying* (in bold), Judy Tatelbaum in *The Courage to Grieve* (in italics), and several chapters of this book (in parentheses).

The stages described by Kübler-Ross, Tatelbaum, and others do not all occur in every grieving situation and are not necessarily experi-

FIGURE 12.1 The Descent

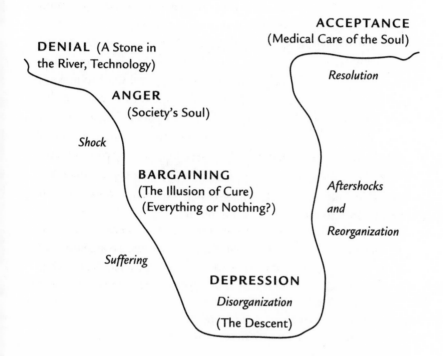

enced in this order. A person may grieve without experiencing a particular stage at all, or may experience a stage more than once in the process. The authors whose works are discussed in the following sections accompany us on this painful but necessary quest.

My Voice Will Go with You

Viktor Frankl, Man's Search for Meaning

In his book, Viktor Frankl recounted the changes he underwent as he was driven ever deeper into the hopelessness of the concentration camps:

> These reactions, as I have described them, began to change in a few days. The prisoner passed from the first to the second phase, the phase

of relative apathy in which he achieved a kind of emotional death. ... And thus the mortification of normal reactions was hastened. ... The sufferers, the dying and the dead, became such commonplace sights to him after a few weeks of camp life that they could not move him anymore.

Several of my colleagues in camp who were trained in psychoanalysis often spoke of a "regression" in the camp inmate—a retreat to a more primitive form of mental life. His wishes and desires became obvious in his dreams.

Under the influence of a world which no longer recognized the value of human life and human dignity, which had robbed man of his will and had made him an object to be exterminated (having planned, however, to make full use of him first—to the last ounce of his physical resources)—under this influence the personal ego finally suffered a loss of values.

I had a distinct feeling that I saw the streets, the squares and houses of my childhood with the eyes of a dead man who had come back from another world and was looking down on a ghostly city.

The prisoners saw themselves completely dependent on the moods of the guards—playthings of fate—and this made them even less human than the circumstances warranted.

The apathy, emotional death, inner retreat, and loss of values experienced by these inmates indicate that they were in denial and shock, and then depressed. Their feelings of helplessness, powerlessness, and numbness removed them from the illusions that had made up their everyday lives.

Thomas Moore, *Care of the Soul*

Care of the soul requires acceptance of all this dying. The temptation is to champion our familiar ideas about life right up to the last second, but it may be necessary in the end to give them up, to enter into the movement of death. If the symptom is felt as the sense that life is over, and that there's no use in going on, then an affirmative approach to this feeling might be a conscious, artful giving-in to the emotions and thoughts of ending that depression has stirred up.

... Cold remorse and self-judgment do not have to be seen as clinical syndromes, but as a necessary foolishness in human life that actually accomplishes something for the soul. ... For the soul, depression is an initiation, a rite of passage. ... Sometimes people need to withdraw and show their coldness. As friends and counselors, we could provide the emotional space for such feelings, without trying to change them or interpret them.

Depression, with its potential for remorse and self-judgment, becomes a rite of passage. Self-examination can reveal meaning and purpose that will form the basis for self-acceptance.

Scott Peck, *Denial of the Soul*

Repeatedly I have used a phrase that is not in general parlance: "the work of depression." Most succinctly it is the work of existential suffering required for the healing of a depression.

But the fact remains, we're likely very miserable, scared, and immobilized, and not one bit grateful for the opportunity to be so. However, as soon as we begin the difficult work of our grief's journey, including slogging through depression, we have begun the road to resolution, acceptance and healing. There is in fact no other way to get there.

Hanging on a Hook

Jean Shinoda Bolen, *Close to the Bone*

Bolen describes the descent of Inanna, the queen of heaven and earth (our consciousness), into the underworld (unconscious):

When Inanna went down through the seven gates into the Great Below, the proud and powerful goddess entered naked and bowed low, looked into the baleful eyes of death, and was struck down. Her body was hung on a hook to rot. She became a slab of green meat. This is a picture of how it feels to be reduced and humbled, powerless and without illusions, to be vulnerable and rejected, to feel putrid. There are phases of being ill in which people feel like Inanna on the hook, when the infected, dysfunctional, or malignant cellular level of their being permeates the soul, and they feel as if they were dead and rotting.

Viktor Frankl, *Man's Search for Meaning*

Former prisoners ... agree that the most depressing influence of all was that a prisoner could not know how long his term of imprisonment would be ... tuberculosis patients in a sanitarium ... also know no date for their release. They experience a similar existence—without a future and without a goal.

I was again conversing silently with my wife, or perhaps I was struggling to find the *reason* for my sufferings, my slow dying ... and from somewhere I heard a victorious "Yes" in answer to my question of the existence of an ultimate purpose.

We who lived in concentration camps can remember the men who walked through the huts comforting others, giving away their last piece of bread ... they offer sufficient proof that everything can be taken from a man but one thing: the last of the human freedoms—to choose one's attitude in any given set of circumstances, to choose one's own way.

A feeling of emptiness is one aspect of depression. It is a dying, a death. When we do the work of letting go of that which has been lost—whether some inner aspect or something or someone without—we begin to fill the empty space with that which is genuine.

Thomas Moore, *Care of the Soul*

In our melancholy, inner construction may be taking place, clearing out the old and putting up the new.

In Saturn, reflection deepens, thoughts embrace a larger sense of time, and the events of a long lifetime get distilled into a sense of one's essential nature.

Depression and grieving are painful work that lead us toward an expansiveness of soul, the generosity of spirit that will nurture acceptance.

Isabel Allende, *Paula*

Winter is back and it won't stop raining; it's cold, and you are worse every day. Forgive me for having made you wait so long, Paula. ... I've been too slow, but now I have no doubt, your letter is so revealing! Count on me, I promise I will help you, just give me a little more time. I sit beside you in the quiet of your room in this winter that will be eternal for me, the two of us alone, just as we have been so often over these months, and I open myself to pain without offering any resistance.

When we are forewarned through their illness of someone's impending death, we have time to prepare in many ways, all of which are aspects of grief. Much of our necessary grieving in this situation is done during the last of the person's life, before death, and is called *anticipatory grief*. Through this process, by the time the death occurs both the dying and those living a bit longer will have completed part of the grieving process.

Fear and avoidance of pain close the door to this passage. What Stephen Levine calls "softening into the pain" or "moving into the pain" gives us access to the deep nature of our spirit that prepares us to heal.

Healing and Ascent

Jean Shinoda Bolen, *Close to the Bone*

Ninshubur, Inanna's devoted friend, carries to the underworld two creatures, one with the nectar of life, the other with the crumbs of the food of life. She arrives at the throne room of Ereshkigal, the enraged, murderous queen of the underworld. She represents our oppressed and buried shadow self; perhaps our very soul.

[The god] told them that they would find Ereshkigal moaning in pain, "with the cries of a woman about to give birth," unclothed, her breasts uncovered and her hair disheveled, and that they were to respond with compassion to her cries.

Each time Ereshkigal moaned in pain, "Oh! Oh! My inside!" they moaned, "Oh! Oh! Your inside!" [*and so forth*] ... and in doing so, they shared and witnessed her pain, until finally, her pain was gone, and she was also no longer the angry, death-bringing baleful goddess. Instead, she was now grateful and generous.

To share and witness each other's pain and experience it is to give a gift. In the search for meaning and purpose, it is invaluable to have others assist by offering compassion and understanding. When we acknowledge fear, anger, depression and entrapment, we help one another move toward acceptance, and beyond.

Viktor Frankl, *Man's Search for Meaning*

Once the meaning of suffering had been revealed to us, we refused to minimize or alleviate the camp's tortures by ignoring them or harboring false illusions and entertaining artificial optimism. Suffering had become a task on which we did not want to turn our backs. We had realized its hidden opportunities for achievement. ...

In spite of all the enforced physical and mental primitiveness of the life in a concentration camp, it was possible for the spiritual life to deepen.

A thought transfixed me: for the first time in my life I saw the truth as it is set into song by so many poets, proclaimed as the final wisdom by so many thinkers. The truth—that love is the ultimate and the highest goal to which man can aspire. ... In a position of utter desolation, when man cannot express himself in positive action, when his only achievement may consist in enduring his sufferings in the right way— an honorable way—in such a position man can, through loving contemplation of the image he carries of his beloved, achieve fulfillment ... soon my soul found its way back from the prisoner's existence to another world, and I resumed talk with my loved one: I asked her questions, and she answered; she questioned me in return, and I answered.

Love goes very far beyond the physical person of the beloved. It finds its deepest meaning in his spiritual being, his inner self. Whether or not he is actually present, whether or not he is still alive at all, ceases somehow to be of importance.

Suffering can be embraced as a catalyst for redefinition of meaning and purpose and can help one move from depression into a vision for the rest of life.

Afterward

Viktor Frankl, *Man's Search for Meaning*

With tired steps we prisoners dragged ourselves to the camp gates. Timidly we looked around and glanced at each other questioningly. Then we ventured a few steps out of camp. This time no orders were shouted at us, nor was there any need to duck quickly to avoid a blow or kick. Oh no! This time the guards offered us cigarettes! We hardly recognized them at first; they had hurriedly changed into civilian clothes. We walked slowly along the road leading from the camp. ... "Freedom"—we repeated to ourselves, and yet we could not grasp it.

... Many days passed, until not only the tongue was loosened, but something within oneself as well; then feeling suddenly broke through the strange fetters which had restrained it. ... "I called to the Lord from my narrow prison and He answered me in the freedom of space."

The crowning experience of all, for the homecoming man, is the wonderful feeling that, after all he has suffered, there is nothing he need fear any more—except his God.

Losses come in many forms. Even this blessed freedom—like the cure of an illness—represented a loss, the loss of what had been, of a period of life lived absolutely without illusions. These men would initially experience denial and undoubtedly would have to work through anger, bargaining, and depression before reaching acceptance of their new, "free" lives.

The descent into grieving and depression strips away the garments by which our mundane existence has hidden us from ourselves. The half-century history of technology is left by the roadside. We turn from society's angry, judgmental voice to something much more genuine, deep within. Dichotomies such as "everything or nothing" reveal themselves to be pale cartoon versions of a much richer mystery. We realize that ultimately we cannot be cured of life but only offered the chance for enlightenment.

Grief is a blessing and the normal, natural response to loss. It is our internal way of working through the terror that loss creates. The work of grieving is painful and may be lengthy, but it is impossible to avoid if we are to remain healthy. It is a tremendous healer, supporter, and catalyst for self-examination, learning, and growth. There is no way to skip the painful aspects of grief, no bridge to carry us over the dark forest of the abyss.

The only way to emerge is to pass through the grief, accepting the sadness, self-questioning, and doubt. The loss must be felt and dealt with in order to be worked through and assimilated into our hearts, our souls, and our stories. Once we've done that, we can concentrate on being grateful for having had that which we have lost. The aftermath of healthy grieving is a new outlook on life and death, an expansiveness of soul, and a being very different from who we were before the journey.

As we traverse the valley, the beasts of illness and death are waiting. We may be devoured by them or we may ride them to places they alone can take us. The things we thought would destroy us become our allies in undertaking "medical care of the soul."

PART FOUR

The River Runs Through Us

*W*hy do the dead walk where I come from? They walk because they are still as important to the living as they were before. They are even more meaningful, as the breadth and depth of our funeral ritual shows. We do not hide their bodies away—because we want to see those bodies to help us remember the person's life and all the good they did for us. We need to remember that they are well on their way to becoming an ancestor. We must see our dead so that we can truly mourn them, all the way through, without restraint, to release the grief from our hearts once and for all.

—Malidoma Somé,
Of Water and the Spirit

THIRTEEN

Medical Care
of the Soul

Finding Our Way to the Soul

Part Three of this book touched on the many ways we avoid but finally are drawn down into the soul work an illness calls us to do. Every year the questions I ask patients change. I've gone from what I should do, to what is needed, to what is wanted, to what is wanting. At the time of this writing I find that all the earlier answers follow from the later questions: What does the soul need or seek to remember in these final, precious minutes or months? And therefore, what should we health care providers do to create the optimal setting for that urgent vision quest? As technicians we ask, "What do I need to do?" A healer must ask, "What have you come here to do? How can I support you so that can happen?"

When I try to remember how my colleagues, my patients, and their families take the first step into that rushing river, it is their eyes that show me the way.

When a person suddenly becomes a patient, his arrival at Admitting labels him with a diagnosis and a proposed treatment procedure. The eyes clearly show fear, even as they also show the hope that they will be cared for somewhere down those sterile halls.

In Critical Care Units, where most Americans will grapple with death, things move quickly. In an hour I've seen the eyes go from jovial to terrified, from stoic to remote. Eyes sparkling with life abruptly close tightly, bracing for the worst. Saddest and most painful

for me are eyes that remain fully aware in a body over which the patient has lost all control—eyes that seem to be looking out from wells
miles deep, as if they've already been sucked into a place far beyond
my reach or the reach of anything else of this world. Those eyes are
so horribly alone, so unprotected. They seem bewildered by what is
happening, without anyone to take the journey with them.

There is an extreme version of brain injury called "locked-in
state" in which the person is awake but unable to move. In many
ways our recoil from the last of life puts us all in a locked-in state,
suspended there within the walls of the Critical Care Unit.

The eyes I most cherish are these same eyes when we call the soul
back from its terror. The call goes something like this: "Here's what
will happen. Here's how your dying will go. Let me tell you what
we're each here to do. We can see to it that your passing will be pain-
less and without fear. But listen: there is still so much you can do for
yourself and your family, and for those of us caring for you, in the
time that remains." The eyes come up out of their tomb; they blink
twice and focus. Discovering around them the very people who have
shared their journey, they reenter the flow of life.

Even as I write this, I become aware of the phrase, "Here's what
we've each come to do." I begin to realize on how many levels those
words can be spoken, and how few of the levels I've usually addressed or even recognized. Viktor Frankl wrote, "But I have to con-
fess here that only too rarely had I the inner strength to make contact with my companions in suffering and that I must have missed
many opportunities for doing so."

My sense is that we bury the soul long before the body gives up.
We discard what this person has to offer in their last moments or
weeks; we shelve what they have been and done for an entire lifetime in order to drag out the heartbeats of a physical entity they
would never have chosen to be.

I wonder about the eyes that go still as we sedate or paralyze a patient to keep him on a ventilator or narcotize him out of his pain.
It's a pharmacologic version of vegetative state, in which brain in-

jury keeps patients alive but in coma for months or decades. What is the soul thinking, experiencing, in these times? What would it tell me if it could? Does it float above the bed, smiling down with a sad compassion for us all? Or does it rail and pound at the rib cage, the tubed belly, the unmoving skull in which it is trapped? Does that soul receive my ministrations as chalices filled with love and honor or as the final horrifying humiliation? When the eyes have gone still, what does this soul have to say? What tasks are left for it to complete? How shall I as a caregiver listen, and how respond?

So many families carry rage or resentment after a death. I believe this reaction is one way in which our patients' souls are crying out to us to be heard, to be cared for, cherished, and honored in a way we do not do now. But what is this "soul" I see looking out at me through my patients' eyes? What qualities give it the right to claim my attention?

Aspects of the Soul

Since scientists work by dissecting the world into its parts, I find myself dividing the soul into four manifestations circumscribed enough for me to understand.

Over the years I've moved from seeing my patients as diseases to seeing them as people, to seeing them as *individual souls*. That is, the rather mundane Western notion of the soul as a distinct, disconnected secular entity. We name this one and encumber her with a Social Security number. She has a medical-record number and insurance policy number, and her chart is closed at the end of the day.

A million steeples and shrines, mosques and sanctuaries evoke the concept of the *eternal* soul. This one came here to do something, to learn or heal old wounds, then to carry back what it experienced. This is the one that some religions say is judged and sent to heaven or hell, or the one that carries the karma of what it did—and had done to it—in each lifetime. This is the one we send packing with a valise full of final papers—adoration and helplessness, hope or dread, pain and courage, defeats that led to beautiful resolutions. If we are in fact reborn and travel through many lives with those we've most touched, I fully expect to be embraced deeply in some instances and brutally mugged in others when I meet my patients the next time around.

My third concept of soul is the *legacy* we leave in this world. This one haunts the families who call in anguish about a loved one's death in the health care system. It lives on in the room where a man used Hospice to help him ease his wife's passing. Since most Americans die in our hospitals, surrounded with our tubes and personnel, we health care providers have remarkable power to shape the legacy a departing soul will leave in this world.

Which brings us to the fourth aspect of soul, which has become steadily more central, more unifying as I've written this book and experienced its impact in my medical practice: the soul as *one*. This is the universal soul that joins us all together.

Come Together

Is there *one* soul that encompasses everything? When we consider such an enormity, we are in the domain of a universal soul that infuses all of us and the cosmos, that joins us and touches us all when even the smallest part is hurt, or trembles, or rejoices. When health care workers move out of our isolation into an intimate experience of our dying patients and those who love them, something opens up in us that had been closed our whole lives.

When we join our patients at the level of soul, we discover to our amazement that we're not alone, playing to a hostile crowd. Our patients rediscover their strength, deep within a newfound center. The families who've battled, been cajoled, convinced, and manipulated, suddenly invite the professional caregivers into their fold. The ancient wisdom and compassion of clergy, Hospice, social workers, and our own pasts and passions converge. And above and behind us, the ancestors, the spirits, the ancients we have welcomed home at last reach in to guide our every step.

FOURTEEN

The Soul's Calling:
Illness as the Way In

Care of the soul sees another reality altogether. It appreciates the mystery of human suffering and does not offer the illusion of a problem-free life. It sees every fall into ignorance and confusion as an opportunity to discover the beast residing at the center of the labyrinth is also an angel. The uniqueness of a person is made up of the insane and twisted as much as it is of the rational and normal. To approach this paradoxical point of tension where adjustment and abnormality meet is to move closer to the realization of our mystery-filled, star-born nature.

—Thomas Moore, *Care of the Soul*

Illness as a Manifestation of Life's Choices

The Illness from Within

Darryl was under hypnosis at an "Alchemical Hypnotherapy Empowerment Weekend." It was a very California sort of thing. Twelve of us attended this young man, sending him good energy and acting roles that came up in his trance. The major thought I couldn't help but send him was, "What in the world am I doing here, and how do I escape gracefully?" My turn was coming; I seriously doubted that anything short of a billy club could put me under.

Darryl was approaching the garden gate behind which lurked the ancient secret that had wrecked his present life. A huge, surly guard in medieval garb blocked his way. Abruptly Darryl cried out for his inhaler—his asthma was tightening up. Instead the hypnotist leading this carnival insisted that he could deal with the attack through imagery. Why was his throat closing? What was blocking him? It was the guard grabbing him by the neck.

The beast could be convinced to become a guide and aid; the hypnotist suggested that Darryl tell him the commandment to shield the gate was from a time long past and no longer helpful. As this suggestion took hold, the young man's wheezing abated and disappeared. And so did mine.

For the past five years, I had been experiencing progressively more severe bouts of bronchitic asthma. It had reached the point of courses of cortisone, which scared me half to death. Every time I tried to speak what was on my mind, I ended up choking and coughing. In over a year, I'd not had a day that I didn't need to use the inhalers just to keep going. Three inhalers were out in my car as I suffocated right along with Darryl. That night, after totally failing to either be hypnotized or fool those in the room into thinking I was, I beat myself up for eight straight hours, straining to figure out what was blocking me. Who were *my* guards from times past? What was choking back my voice and my will? How did I get myself into these ridiculous situations anyway?

By morning, I'd realized that the ridiculous situation haunting me was not the weekend, but rather my life. I had believed, and confirmed over and over, that the only way I could hold my life together was by accepting bad contracts—work 120 hours per week and pretend to be happy, give more than I could and feel used in return, live without passion or safety but pretend such a life was okay. All the time, I was choking back my raging desire to scream, "This stinks; this isn't fair; this isn't who I was meant to be!" Clamping my trachea closed. Stifling the scream. Then having more rage leak out in a dozen dysfunctional ways that screwed up my life even more.

On my return home, I began speaking what was on my mind, and then things really went to hell in a handbasket. In the rather difficult year since, I've had not one moment of bronchospasm. I'm "cured," not by a medication that took away the symptom but by seeing the metaphor, the misconceptions at the root of the illness.

First among our list of inalienable rights are those of "life, liberty, and the pursuit of happiness." Unfortunately, nobody warned us how many choices these rights entail and how many different scripts underlie both what we choose and how we interpret the consequences of our choices. According to the judgmental, blaming mode described in Chapter 9, "When Society's Soul Speaks," my asthma was a "self-induced illness." I'd chosen jobs and situations that demanded more of me than I could give. I'd made unrealistic promises, stretched myself to the breaking point, all in hopes of being found worthy of love and approval. Yet my resentment of "their" demanding so much caused me to act in ways that had the opposite effect. I was irritable. I was reactive. I was "leaking" misplaced and inappropriate frustrations like crazy.

It was my view of my place in the world and of what I had to do to survive that had distorted my relations to others. My projection of how "they" judged me then magnified the negative reactions I got from others, and my responses became as misdirected, inappropriate, and huge as those of any lumbering fairy-tale giant.

And I did what as a child I'd concluded was all I could do to hold it together—choke back the truth.

My kind of medicine pictures asthma as an inflammatory condition of the airways with immunologic, genetic, environmental, and emotional components. We know that emotions modulate the immune and endocrine systems. We picture emotions as nerve endings releasing endorphins, catecholamines, and dopaminergic mediators that affect smooth-muscle contractility. But is the emotional component something much deeper? Are we inflamed by the outrage of our soul at its neglect? Does it recognize how suffocating and airless is the environment our egos have constructed in pursuit of power and false safety? Are we rejecting ourselves, attempting to cough out the disease we've drawn into our lives?

An environmental ecologist might say I should move to Arizona, cultivate kumquats, and lead a quiet life. In an opposing view, James Hillman's *We've Had a Hundred Years of Psychotherapy and the World Is Getting Worse* warned that we've become so focused on our individual plights and "inner children" that we've lost the societal context of why we should get straightened out in the first place. I believe, like Alcoholics Anonymous and many others, that the individual cure must be manifested in outward service and activity.

The issue of causality also affects how we interpret a dis-ease. Many illnesses, like my asthma, may be at least in part self-induced. When we ask, "Why me? Why did this illness befall me?" perhaps we should really ask, "Why did my soul choose this particular illness to make me look at my life?" If, as Hillman suggested, the "Soul's Code" knows what we're here to do, then illness becomes one of the most powerful ways for the soul to get our attention, stop us in our tracks, turn us on a dime, and make us listen. Then speak. Then do.

As we tend to feel that illness comes from something outside ourselves, we often feel victimized by the circumstances around us that force illness upon us. But is this an instance of the world muffling the potential of our soul or of our soul using circumstances to reach toward its purpose?

Carrying the Illness for Those Nearest to Us

Some illnesses are what I would call socially induced. I've seen entire families focus for years or decades on the one member who is sick or developmentally delayed, self-abusing, or dying. In such cases, a great deal of love, commitment, and compassion becomes attached to the central figure and his or her problem. But that individual carries a heavy burden, and so much has been invested in a structure with that illness at its core that if the illness goes away or the person dies, nobody knows what to do. Renal transplantation as a treatment for end-stage renal disease has been singularly unsuccessful in preventing divorce or re-creating employability. When the cancer is "cured," we may discover it was distracting us from something else eating at the social structure around the survivor. Jerome Groopman in *The Measure of Our Days* described a man who became despondent when his renal-cell carcinoma went into remission. He concluded that his family "will be fine without me. ... The remission meant nothing because it was too late to relive my life. I once asked for hell. Maybe God made this miracle to have me know what it will feel like." His tumor had manifested the sickness at the core of his life and had offered him the chance to escape it without dealing with his inability to feel love.

In these settings, the soul of the individual sings in the larger chorus of the soul of the family. How are individuals perceived and valued? What is missing, what is aching to heal or be healed by the family? What darkness is being denied? What does the individual's suffering illuminate for those she loves and turns to for love? What strength screams out to be tested, felt, proven in this deep womb of relationship?

Perhaps we are all necessarily sacrificed. Each of us has given up or buried something precious just to make it through our days. The question is not what was taken from me but what I gave away, what my soul arranged through illness to have stripped from me, that I might find the deeper truth in myself.

Spiritually Induced Illness

We are in a time of radical fundamentalism in Islam, Christianity, Judaism, and some animist faiths. All proclaim how deeply something is missing. In *Care of the Soul*, Thomas Moore wrote,

> The vague emotional complaints of our time, complaints we therapists hear every day in our practice, include:
>
> emptiness
> meaninglessness
> vague depression
> disillusionment about marriage, family and relationship
> a loss of values

yearning for personal fulfillment
a hunger for spirituality

All of these symptoms reflect a loss of soul and let us know what the soul craves.

Scott Peck proposed in *Denial of the Soul* that the demand for active euthanasia is one final secular attempt to maintain control over one's own body, denying that we belong to anything but ourselves, that we're connected to anything else, or that our suffering could have any purpose beyond the point of our physical existence.

Illness seems to both challenge and evoke our spiritual side. "How could this happen to me?" "What good is my faith if it offers nothing now when my mother is sick?" "I'm nothing now that I can't work." "I don't want to be a burden on my family." "It's all hopeless, hopeless." I've seen lifelong churchgoers absolutely bleak and isolated when facing death. I've seen entrenched atheists radiant with peace and revelation as they approach the end. Like the Inquisition's trial by fire, illness and approaching death hold us up to the flame, burn away the dross. They introduce the saint in us to the witch.

Yet our soul is more witch than saint: it is deeply connected to earth and to our bodies, to death and to mystery. It works spells in the way we reveal our malaise and our potential in our body's signs. It speaks incantations in the words that grab our minds when illness makes all else irrelevant. If it reveals just how little we are connected to our spiritual force, it also offers the chance to heal that split. If it clarifies what truly, deeply, eternally has meaning to us—be it God or our children, truth or the scent of a flower in a vase by the window, a puppy curled at our feet or a well-turned phrase—then we discover our soul seeking to heal us of our own lifelong isolation from ourselves.

What does this illness call me to face? Am I enslaved by outdated beliefs? The soul calls me to hold my presumptions in my hands for closer inspection. Odds are, they'll slip away like sand being swept out to sea. Are the choices that once saved me now destroying me?

It's time to consider which doors those choices closed, and through which others I now must pass.

Is it my place in the family or my professional role that no longer "works"? What "essential" quality of myself is illness calling me to discard like an outdated pair of bell-bottom pants?

Can I no longer accept the strictures and prejudices my society has imposed upon me, which I accepted because I believed they reflected who I was? My soul may be telling me I've been brought here to see, to name, and to challenge the illness in my society's soul.

What will I do with this malaise of my and all our spirits that makes my life and death meaningless? My illness is offering to draw back the veils of illusion so I may at last feel the true fire and ice deep within me and my world. Whatever illness or death drew you to a book like this was the manifestation of your soul declaring that it would be ignored no longer.

This Body Through Which the Soul Speaks

Drawing on ancient, through Renaissance, to contemporary sources, Thomas Moore described the human body as

> an immense source of imagination, a field on which the imagination plays wantonly. ... Therefore, a poetic reading of the body as it expresses itself in illness calls for a new appreciation for the laws of imagination, in particular a willingness to let imagination keep moving into ever newer and deeper insights. ... The object of therapeutic treatment is to return imagination to things that have become only physical. ... A specialist in disease should begin his questions for diagnosis with issues of pleasure. Are you enjoying life? Where is it not pleasurable? Are you fighting pleasure? The history of philosophy demonstrates the remarkable fact that whenever soul is placed at the center of concern, pleasure is one of the most prominent factors discussed.

This "immense field on which imagination plays" has been perceived and responded to in countless ways. And of course, what we expect to find, we find. A running theme of Stephen Jay Gould's column, "A View of Life," in *Natural History* magazine is that our presumptions about the world determine what questions we ask and how we interpret the answers. The great physicist Heisenberg showed that the act of observation itself changes the outcome of what is observed. *So all our views of the body and of illness are models that support our presumptions about what makes up reality.* I want to touch on some of these interpretations because each may offer some way of understanding what goes "wrong" or "right" in our relationship to our bodies and their ills.

The Machine

Our "science," which means "knowing," implies that there is only one truth and that that truth is neither "good" nor "bad." In this view, we are intricate but ultimately knowable machines with no dimension beyond the physical. Emotions are variations in level and receptors for dopamine, catecholamines, and other chemical messengers. We jog or get tattoos to stimulate morphinelike endorphins. Aging is a process of the machine breaking down: call in the mechanics. The heart is a pump, the liver is a chemical factory, and our kidneys are mere sieves designed to keep nephrologists like myself in business.

The metaphor is that illness occurs because of rust, poor maintenance, faulty design, or inevitable wear and tear. Physicians should identify the worn part, adjust or replace it, and get this little beauty back on the road. When the body becomes sufficiently unserviceable, park it on the back-lot nursing home until it rots away. Larry Dossey emphasized in *Meaning and Medicine* that such a mechanistic view devoid of meaning leaves us with "no intent in our life— no activity or energy, no goal to pursue. With no story to tell, no purpose, and no activity, we are as good as dead." Scientific medicine has done a terrific job of salvaging the machine. In some cases we've even grudgingly pushed the owners to do preventive maintenance. But our steadfast refusal to consider meaning or imagination in illness limits both our diagnostics and our therapeutics. The heart is no longer the seat of emotions and character but a muscular pump. The mind is paramount, which is kind of funny since it's got fewer moving parts than anything but the kidneys. Even fingernails are more dynamic than the all-powerful mind!

A friend of mine has a port-wine hemangioma, a purple birthmark, covering much of his right foot. For years it was just there. Then one day it started weeping, literally shedding tears. A specimen was taken that not only was misinterpreted as cancer but left a wound that would not heal. With the misdiagnosis and the ulceration, I count two wounds that would not heal. To doctors like me, such vascular malformations are a simple matter of hydraulics, oxygen metabolism, and inflammation. There was too much back-pressure in the receiving veins, too much blood heating the tissues too much. The red cells, inflammatory cells, and proteins that should have been lovingly soothing his tissues were instead consuming them. My technologic recommendation would have been to blow open the veins, irradiate the abnormal channels, and suppress the inflammatory response. We no longer turn to the Madonna of Lourdes for divine revelation. This was a gummed-up pipe, and we should have blown the thing open.

The scientific metaphor by definition precludes the soul. When intellect reaches down like the hand of some wrathful Jehovah to eliminate purpose and intent, to sweep away all the darkness and mystery, it slays the soul. When the soul tries to reach us through the screens of our mechanistic interpretation, it is like a prisoner throwing tiny pebbles through his bars at the Sphinx. He doesn't exist.

Energy Blockages

Acupuncture sees the body as a vibrant energy network with illness and its cure based on blockages that emotion, injury, or other factors place in the way of the healthy flow. The needles "realign" the energy flux. Reikke therapy, meditative visualization, and some spiritual healing practices add the concept that a beautiful energy suffuses us, moving down from the cosmos through the top of our heads

(Seventh Chakra) or up from the earth (First Chakra). When we open up, or a Reikke therapist opens us up, to this energy, we're filled with almost limitless potential for strength and healing. When we're blocked, we're cut off and weakened.

This perspective is nearly the opposite of the material view that founds my science. Yet the two converge at the molecular and atomic levels, where energy and matter become inseparable. At the microneuroanatomic level, thought evolves a network of ever-branching dendrites, chemical modifications, and discharges more dizzying than any celestial circus. In my science, I know that a cancer will devour all the nutrition I can offer my patient. It's eating him, draining her from within. I call it nutritional deprivation. Others would say it's consuming his energy, drawing energy away from the rest of the body, shutting off access to the healing energy of earth and heaven.

Is it true? Is it good? Who of us hasn't felt drained of energy, in need of having our batteries recharged? When I turn on myself in rage or despair, arthritis or cancer, am I shorting out through channels demonically connected? When I'm energized by a relationship, by love or revelation, do I draw my energy from imagination or from some celestial or deeply earthy source? Or do I drag it out of my companion in an endless act of mutual cannibalism?

What blockage of energy is being manifested by the fatty plaques that fill my arteries? What desperate holding on contorts my bowels and plugs me up like a blocked piece of plumbing? How is it that music, meditation, love, prayer, and camping deep in the mystery-laden mountains have identical impacts on our "vital signs"?

My friend's foot continues to fester. The acupuncturist says he's shut off energy to it, that he has to accept it back into his body, love it, that the blockage of energy is preventing healing. Not being a podiatrist, I have a distinctly hard time imagining loving more than one or two of the feet I've known. But my friend can feel a specific point of pain when his acupuncturist works, and a surge ascends his leg just before the swelling starts to recede. As that surge moves toward his head, he feels the beginning of hope, of acceptance and joy. When he describes the sensation, I can almost hear his soul take in a deep breath and begin unfolding itself into an upright, upstanding position.

Herbs, Homeopathy, and the American Pharmaceutical Association

We are chemical entities, and our illnesses are deficiencies or excesses of chemicals that can be reformulated. My brother believes our entire clan has a hereditary deficiency in dopamine receptors, leading to "reward deficiency syndrome." Sounds right to me, though I think our behavior is all learned. Perhaps we're both right: if we never learn how to feel joy and reward, perhaps we never lay down the dopaminergic dendrites, the behavior patterns, the ways of perceiving that would reinforce rewardable behaviors and peacefulness. As an internist, herbs and drugs make perfect sense to me.

Homeopathy draws a bit on the ancient notion that the god or agent that caused the illness carries its cure. Practitioners of this ephemeral religion dilute some toxic stuff so far that there's "not one molecule left," only the "essence" or "spirit." Now here I am writing a book to say that if we neglect the scientifically nonexistent soul, all of our physical efforts are pointless at best, evil at worst. Yet homeopathy is a stretch for me. Could be, though. When we imbibe any of this stuff, whether it's Saint-John's-wort for a buck and a half, a vial labeled "cantharis" full of highly spirited water, or a cephalosporin antibiotic 150 times as precious as gold on the open market, placebo effect makes up 40 to 80 percent of the benefit. So clearly there are more players on the field than just exogenous chemicals banging against nerve end-plates.

Metaphorically, I'm sure life is chock-full of deficiencies, excesses, and deceitful messengers bearing false witness. I'm "down a quart," "playing with half a deck," "hot under the collar." I "can't get no satisfaction," am "hot and bothered," "inflamed," "rotten to the core," and just plain "eating myself up inside." That's just me, not to mention the rest of the world! The question is whether the cure lies in killing the culprit or in listening to the twining metaphors of the vessel that would speak through its illness.

My friend with the bum foot tries herbs to encourage wound healing, applies serum extracts directly on the wound, uses homeopathy to treat the inflammation with the stigmata of inflammation, and eats well and lives a good life. The sores continue crying their eyes out as his own eyes remain dry. But because he's hurting and because the wound is visible, his soul has called him to tend to himself, to seek his own healing. And the missteps and outright screwups of my kind of medicine have driven him directly into the calling of his own soul.

The Organs Speak

Thomas Moore described his colon complaining and paining over its lack of "organ eroticism." Scott Peck and pretty much every other writer in this arena have gone at length into a discussion of depression as a time of healing, change, introspection, awareness, emptying out, reaction to societal denial, Saturn's calling, or (seldom admitted) a pain in the butt. Having experienced the gracious gifts of depression, I'd have to say that all this glorious prose sounds somewhat like a sales pitch for a lovely piece of swamp land in the Everglades.

And how did the "butt" get such a bad rap, anyway? In dream work, when shit appears you're getting down to something real, genuine, profound. Leave it to us to malign the part of our anatomy that squats closest to Mother Earth.

Still, each of us knows exactly where in our bodies we feel angry or contorted when rage, depression, grief, love, or terror rips open the Tupperware containers in which we hide. From reading the future in the entrails of sheep to diagnosing distant illnesses in the ten qualities of the pulse, we admit that organs speak. Our language redounds with ancient and subliminal connections—inspiration, heartfelt, venting your spleen, of like mind, dysthymia, degenerative joints, a rash decision.

Even my kind of medicine has been forced to acknowledge that emotions have something to do with the immune system and those diseases in which we lambaste ourselves. These include such autoimmune diseases (that is, when our immune system attacks rather than defends us) as rheumatoid arthritis, lupus, Crohn's disease, ulcers, heart failure, and cancer. And emotions may well determine the probability of a cure. Some of the best predictors of survival from a severe illness include having pets or underage children at home, support structures, a sense of purpose, and a good outlook on life.

A few of the hundreds of connections from Louise Hay's book, *You Can Heal Your Life*, suggest some of these organ or illness metaphors, as shown in Table 14.1.

Hay's list goes on for sixty-one more pages, from blackheads to zits. Now, as far out as some of this may seem, I've discovered that when I let myself go, shoot from the hip (not far from Second Chakra, the generative center), and spout out whatever metaphor comes to mind with my patients, I nearly always hit the mark and always stir up something of value. When I encountered a man dying of unexplained repeated gastrointestinal bleeding, he said he was terrified of dying, yet his eyes seemed far away and glazed over with indifference. I asked him if he was really afraid or if something in him actually wanted to die. At first he looked outraged, then confused, then caught red-handed (again, a bloody good metaphor). Yes, he admitted, he wanted the suffering to be over. What suffering? All of his remorse since he'd discovered his forty-year-old daughter dead of a heart attack. When I told him he didn't have to die to get back to her, that she could come into this world to guide and comfort him, the bleeding stopped. I don't know what happened after that. I was just weekend coverage in one point of a long life. But I do believe that for one moment we were in the presence of the soul crouching behind those glassy eyes.

Recently I informed a beautiful, gentle man that he was dying of melanoma. His diabetes had led to cardiac disease, which led to a heart transplant. Following several surgeries for vascular disease, the

TABLE 14.1 Health Problems, Probable Causes, and New Thought Patterns

Problem	Probable Cause	New Thought Pattern
Abscess	Fermenting thoughts over hurts, slights, and revenge	I allow my thought to be free. The past is over. I am at peace.
Alcoholism	"What's the use?" Feeling of futility, guilt, inadequacy. Self-rejection.	I live in the now. Each moment is new. I choose to see my self-worth. I love and approve of myself.
Allergies	Who are you allergic to? Denying your own power.	The world is safe and friendly. I am safe. I am at peace with life.
Asthma	*Smother* love. Inability to breathe for one's self. Feeling stifled. Suppressed crying.	It is safe now for me to take charge of my own life. I choose to be free.
Birth Defects	Karmic. You selected to come that way. We choose our parents and our children. Unfinished business.	Every experience is perfect for our growth process. I am at peace with where I am.

requisite immunosuppression unleashed his body's tendency to form tumors, which will now take him away. It's a story of bad luck and iatrogeny—illness induced by medical treatment. If "the God who wounds is the God who can cure," we must also recognize that he who would be a healer can and often does also wound. Or in metaphoric terms it could go like this: something in him attacked his pancreas, which caused all the excess of sweetness in his life to

pile up in his vital passages. What was nutritious and flowing became mortally clogged. He lost heart—but by turning to the genie
of technology was born anew—but each request of the genie is answered not quite in the way we sought and anticipated. There's a
trick to each prize. The blockages in his body spread out of control,
and his body's desire to expand, to be released, won. Now the dark
places in him will prevail over what any of us attempt to do to "cure"
him. They fill his mind, they close his throat, they consume every
drop of his energy. His cells' lust for life is awakening and will no
longer be turned away.

We delayed his death, and I'm deeply grateful that we could do
so for such a wonderful man. But in the end, the soul will speak, one
way or another, and finally we have no choice but to listen.

When I visited my friend, he was clunking around on his bad foot,
running off to his various jobs, returning to cook meals for his house
full of kids and dependents, coordinating more contracts and sport-
ing events, and building an addition for more family members to
move into. I know he came from a very difficult and somewhat solitary childhood, with a family that gave him considerable reason to
pursue the hermit's life. I asked him if he thought the loads he was
carrying had anything to do with his foot's complaint. He said he
was sure not, and quickly changed the topic.

I think we each could stand to play with metaphor, attempt to
hear what our organs might be trying to tell us through our dis-eases.
Maybe that's why those huge monstrosities with pipes and bellows
belting out the polyphonic howlings of the gods tromping over the
squashy heads of devils are called "organs." The soul never speaks in
simple monosyllables.

Karma

The last column of Louise Hay's list gets me back to the trouble I
have with the notion of "empowering" or "blaming" the individual
for his or her fate. I remain unconvinced that the beautiful children
I saw dying in Sudan sat in the spirit world and decided, "It would

be a great learning experience for me to go down to earth and starve and rot for three years and die." Maybe so, but one would think celestial beings could make better choices.

On the other hand, Brian Weiss's books, *Only Love Is Real* and *Many Lives, Many Masters*, not only drove me green with envy over their nifty titles but convinced me that we probably do come around again and again and again. The spear wound in the shoulder, the rape in a time of war, the heroic death in the plague may indeed be manifested in this life as a painful arm, reproductive troubles, or remarkably good health. Perhaps the children abandoned and unpardonable crimes committed in another time can be atoned for only if we experience abandonment by others and hopelessness now. Did Philoctetes, wounded in the right heel, came back with a port-wine stain that weeps 2,500 years later in a California suburb?

So much seems inexplicable. Science declares that's either because a thing doesn't exist or because we haven't done the right experiment. Brian Weiss's well-documented work with psychotherapy patients under hypnosis makes me suspect we see so little because we refuse to consider so much. His first book, *Many Masters, Many Lives*, documented the gradual conversion of a traditionally trained psychiatrist not at all interested in past-life experiences. Then a series of hypnosis sessions with one client took them both back to the time at which her phobias developed—back into prior lives. The information she and her "Masters" gave to Dr. Weiss made a skeptic into a believer. With that change in viewpoint, his entire life was changed.

Unless we take the additional leap of believing that all past and future lives happen simultaneously and that what we do now affects all, we're forced to leap instead to the question, "So, what's the point? Why the devil would an omnipotent and benign patriarchal god make me suffer now for something I already suffered for back then, and can't undo anyway?"

The answer is an extension of our current mythology called psychology. We can accept that we're wounded in childhood and may keep reenacting those woundings until we learn to heal them. Perhaps some of our dis-eases are even more ancient wounds looking to be healed. The rapist in another life is raped in this, learning empathy and loss. The mother who abandoned her children in a past life is given up for adoption this time; her new parents divorce; she is rejected in love. Finally through an illness she encounters the true power and beauty of her connection to dozens, hundreds, of others who love her.

In dreams, in reverie, or in storytelling we can relive either the memory or the metaphor of where this pain was born and how to put it to rest. We should be concerned not so much about what is "true" as about what is "good," which in itself is the healing.

There is another aspect to the soul working in the area of karma. Thomas Moore quoted Paul Tillich, from *The Courage to Be:* "Man is split within himself. Life moves against itself through aggression, hate, and despair. We are wont to condemn self-love; but what we really mean to condemn is contrary to self-love. It is that mixture of selfishness and self-hate that permanently pursues us, that prevents us from loving others, and that prohibits us from losing ourselves in the love with which we are loved eternally. ... But the depth of our separation lies in just the fact that we are not capable of a great and merciful divine love towards ourselves."

The soul doesn't deal in straight lines, simple opposites, or pat answers. Its workroom is filled with mirrors. Shadow and sleight-of-hand abound. Our abuse of others abuses ourselves: perhaps we come here to experience overtly what was unspeakably secret before. We are victim and victimizer alike: Do we repeat to remember the other role we denied having played? My enemy, myself. My illness that will cure me of my illusion of sickness.

The Soul's Calling!

In *The Soul's Code*, James Hillman recounted a popular story of Manolete, *el supremo* of Spanish bullfighters, destined to die in the ring at thirty-two years of age. As a boy, he was "tied to his mother's apron strings," timid and withdrawn, literally hiding behind her apron. At thirteen, a teacher, a guide, a guru of cutting the bull down to size found the boy, and from that moment on his fate was sealed. Traditionally, the story is viewed as an overly macho reaction to shame about cowardliness as a boy. Hillman suggested (in a view that dates back at least to Aristotle) that the opposite was true: that the soul comes into this world knowing what it's here to experience, that it arranges events and our interpretation of them so as to achieve its ends. If you knew subconsciously, Hillman asked, that one day you would find yourself in vast arenas facing two thousand–pound bulls with bad attitudes and sharp horns, wouldn't you hide behind your mother's skirt?

When the soul calls, the message and the messenger may be utterly incomprehensible. In the vernacular of fairy tales, we don't know if this mysterious visitation is the wizened little man at the roadside who holds the keys to adventure and salvation or the evil wizard disguised as a fair maiden, here to distract us from our path. In describing the "wizard's" sense of the "ally," Carlos Castaneda answered this dichotomy with a resounding "yes." The ally is both the wild energy that threatens to destroy and elude us and the benefactor whose challenge, if accepted, will release our deepest potential.

For better or worse, most of us live our lives wrapped in layer upon cellophane layer of assumed safety and insurance forms, bills to be paid, month after endless month. Illness and the brush with death are two of the winds that most drive the soul's voice through the sedating effects of our modern lives. The problem is first to accept the message and then to ferret out the calling in all its mysterious, ambivalent poetry.

Consider the "deathbed" scene of the family and caregivers arrayed around an individual who is battling an illness. Everyone in that small scenario has been called, each in different ways, to bear witness to their own souls and follow their echoing cries. Each will hear a different message and be offered the chance to attend to a different aspect of the needed healing. But for the vast majority, all we will hear is our own grief-stricken fears crying, "Why, Father, have you abandoned me?"

Hearing the Soul's Call

Dreams

The more terrifying their content, the more dreams want us to listen. They may be filled with tarantulas that turn into shoe clerks and beautiful women who have come to kill us. They trap us in eternally reenacting the worst parts of our lives, each time sampling a slightly different twist. They offer amazing resolutions to conflicts and elysian fields of uncharted bliss. In such scoundrelly and contradictory terms does the soul speak.

Fairy Tales

Fairy tales are great and ancient windows on the soul. They instruct us: "Get down off your high horse, let go of the reins of your presumptions, and listen to the little man at the roadside. He may look so ridiculous you'll just boot him into the gutter, but not half as ridiculous as you will returning home without horse, reins, boots, glory, or kingdom." Illness is a great way to get us off our high horse.

Redemption Stories

Shortly after the horrors of Dachau, Buchenwald, Hiroshima, and Nagasaki, Heinrich Zimmer came out with a remarkable book titled *The King and the Corpse: Tales of the Soul's Conquest of Evil*. While I'm sure it has a hundred themes I missed altogether, the one that stood out for me was that to conquer evil, to fight it, even to face it, we must first recognize and act out the evil that is in us. Fifty years later Mary Ciofolo, a gifted therapist in San Francisco, is completing a book of "redemption stories," this time not ancient myths and religious tracts but the stories of contemporary lives. These fifty people have been deeply wounded and scarred. They were party to great evils or transgressions but turned the unforgivable toward healing themselves and the world. The prototype of my profession is Aescu-lapius, the "wounded healer" whose efforts led to his son's death and whose guilt guided his compassion and his hand the rest of his days.

In essence, this entire book is a redemption story: how one physi-cian's career might offer something back to all he has wounded or healed and by whom he has been wounded or made whole; how each death can redeem the life of which it is a part.

Shamanic Journeys

Our wounds, our abuses, our darkness cut us to our core. Revealed, we may disseminate our sickness far and wide or transform into a benediction what has hurt for so long. Illness is for the patient, the family, and the caregivers as close as most of us will get to a shaman's journey. We become intoxicated, altered, dysfunctional. What is normal in us, even our flesh and consciousness, falls away. We go down into the darkness, where we grapple with terrifying, ill-formed, immense forces. We decompose.

And that is where most of us stop in our modern brush with ill-ness and death.

But the journey is meant to continue: the spirits that sought to destroy us become our guides, our allies, our totem animals. We re-turn altered to the world of light. We know the name and meaning of the cure. We bring new blessing into this aging world.

Nowadays we are reluctant to give ourselves fully to our grief and terror because we dread the pain and certain devastation of the first half of the journey. But if we accept it and descend into it as de-scribed in Chapter 12, "The Descent," the second half of the jour-ney is the crucible in which our soul transforms itself from lead into gold. The outcome has the potential to enrich the ones we love and the part of ourselves, our hidden soul, that cries out to be known.

The Vision Quest

In Chapter 17, "The Soul as Legacy," I'll touch on the desire to cre-ate how we will be remembered. This concept applies not just to the patient. Everyone in the room is hoping to lay down a memory—a powerful tale, a handprint on the cave's wall—that will ennoble and clarify his or her own soul's journey. We can look at our minutes and months at the bedside as some huge gridlock, a grotesque speed bump in the highway of life, some endless line waiting to get a burger at the window of salvation. But we can just as well see this as the landscape where a vision quest is opening up before us. We are called to turn toward tasks that have been postponed far too long. I can tell you I'm terrible at this. I'm trained by profession and inclination to spend about five minutes per day at a patient's bedside. When I've had relatives in the hospital, I get itchy at about four and a half minutes. Gotta run. Gotta go check the chart. Time to move on. The soul's rearing head feels like a huge gas bubble in my belly, crying out to get belched.

So I run before something escapes me. I never get around to opening the book to the first picture of that long, arduous, and unnerving quest for vision. But it's there before me nevertheless. The rare times that I didn't flee, the journey touched me to my core. Oh, so that's what it's like to love someone more deeply than yourself after sixty years of marriage. Now I recognize that beautiful, graceful child cowering and vibrantly alive inside the hide of that burned-out addict. Hmm, so that's what it feels like when I stop recoiling from being touched.

We should open ourselves to our dreams and their clearest voices, which are our nightmares. We should share the most absurd thoughts and images that this illness, this weird setting, has brought to mind. We should learn to treasure the haunting presence of the soul's tricksters and their skillful, hidden hands in the room.

Humor

As a child, I quickly learned that the only way I could get away with shining a light on the skeletons in my family's closet was by making a joke. They could blow it off; they could laugh; they could ignore it. But every joke that works has one foot in reality and one foot in mystery. "Laugh therapy," comic relief after the heaviest point in the drama, Hopi contraries—all are examples of the soul poking its festooned head out of the weighty swamp of life.

I've made some terrible jokes in moments of great tragedy and seriousness. When we are truly present for the last of a life, we remember not just the profound and laudable; the profane and laughable are perhaps even more likely to touch our hearts. We may honor Dad's diligence and his struggles, his losses and his pains. But to remember the time he said, "Now, this may be a little damp," before sinking up to his armpits in a swamp takes us back to a time we were all together, immortal, weightless. We need to tell the departing loved one how much we will miss him or her. But some part of us also needs to clear away the old resentments and disappointments. For that, little beats a shared laugh.

There's little in this world sillier than how we handle the last of life. Either we're eternal, and all this focus on prolonging physical life is pointless unless we use the time well, or we're purely physical, and we should enjoy the last of our time as hedonistically as possible. Religion and humor are inseparable. "Borscht Belt" humor is a proximate extension of rabbinic morality tales. Jesus' band of twelve misfits and scoundrels revealed the greatness at the core of the common man and woman. Zen koans often make us laugh as they mystify us. And Mohammed had a great sense of humor in some of the stories he told: "Should I trust in Allah or tether my camel? You should trust in Allah. And tether your camel." Dare I recall the humorous pratfalls that endeared this woman to me, or is this a time of great seriousness? Yes.

Religion

Religion is something of a double-edged sword. Thomas Moore in *Care of the Soul* captured the difference between pursuit of the spirit and pursuit of the soul: "The soul is, as Jung says, the 'archetype of life,' embedded in details of ordinary, everyday experience. In the spirit, we try to transcend our humanity; in the soul, we try to enter our humanity fully and realize it completely." Moore later stated,

> Deep education entails an emergence of character and personality, and often takes the form of initiation. In this sense, a person can be educated by the death of a relative or a friend, as, in one of the earliest recorded tales, the proud Gilgamesh was educated and profoundly transformed by witnessing the death of his friend Enkidu. To be educated, a person doesn't have to know much or be informed, but he or she does have to have been exposed vulnerably to the transformative events of an engaged life. ... Eternal ideas, beauty of expression, a concern for values, and a human scale all give education a soul and soul an education. ... Without an education, the heart presents itself as a cauldron of raw emotions, suspicious desires, and disconnected images.

James Hillman in *We've Had a Hundred Years of Therapy and the World is Getting Worse*, "associates the soul with beauty and death." Beauty, death, "love, desire, and pleasure": are we speaking of the loftiest of human longings, for God and the eternal, or the most intimate, for that which is most physical and shadowy in ourselves? Again, as with all questions about the mysterious soul, the answer is yes.

I have seen religious belief sustain and direct the dying in the most beautiful of ways. But I've also seen these beliefs used as an escape from the dark messages and potential healings the last of life can bring. I've seen those unsupported by religion collapse into the utter meaninglessness of their time on this earth, but just as often I've seen their unrestricted souls carry them to a true religious enlightenment. At worst, the different urges of soul and spirit finalize the split our culture feels between the clean, bright airiness of God and the jumbled, sweaty heaviness of the body.

But at their best, soul and spirit are inseparable companions— Quixote and Sancho Panza, the Lone Ranger and Tonto, Jack Benny and his fiddle. You can fiddle all you want, but if you won't accept the screeches and scratches, you'll never play heaven's lofty arabesques.

I suspect that the most profound religion has its feet set deep in the very fleshy grape vat of the soul. Without an eye to some sort of eternal, the cosmic, a god whose presence gives purpose to our suffering, it's hard to find the courage to truly face the soul's demands.

Listening

As Scott Peck and Stephen Levine have emphasized, pain isn't just a symptom to be put away. It's some part of ourselves calling to be attended to. Going into the pain, we can hear the message. "Softening" into the pain, inviting it in, we can come to peace with what is hurting in us. Going toward rather than away from our existential pains, we can learn what in us cries out to be honored while we're still here to do it. "Doing everything," as the phrase is used in the hospital, describes doing everything to beat back the illness but nothing whatsoever to move into it or learn from it. "We did everything we could." No, in terms of meaning and honoring the soul, we abandoned our patient altogether.

FIFTEEN

The Soul as Individual:
I Will Pass This
Way Only Once

*"My mom's breathing was different, her face was changing. I held
her in my arms to get her head up higher. She died with me holding
her. I can hardly believe it has happened. I remember her telling me
of the time she was with her mother as she died. She held her, too."
The nurse, who was listening intently to this amazing story of how
several generations of mothers and daughters experienced birth and
death together, each in their own turn, suddenly realized who else
was standing in the bedroom area next to the body. It was the
granddaughter of the woman who had just died. Each woman stood
in a circle in awe of the miracle of life and death and of the presence
of generations of family past, present and future.*

—Jan Bernard and Miriam Schneider,
The True Work of Dying

The Concept of the Individual

A great contradiction lies at the core of American, perhaps all Western, psyches. No other culture has so institutionalized, romanticized,
and been enslaved by the concept of the individual. We consider the
individual and his or her rights, history and potential as separate
from any connection to the community of which he or she is a part.

America's outcome may well be a test of one hypothesis: that the individual's needs are best served by guaranteeing individual rights without responsibilities.

As I mentioned in Chapter 7, our ethical principles are pretty much a full house for the individual. Yet here's the contradiction: we're also a society that espouses the belief that all individuals are (created) equal, that everyone should receive health care whether they can pay or not, and that payer status or lifestyle should not be considered in what services are provided. So I'm supposed to see the uniqueness of my patient but ignore almost everything that makes him unique. He was shot in a drug deal? Patch him up! He hates his life and is in constant pain? So what? She has no support but feeds the pigeons and is dearly loved in the neighborhood? Irrelevant. He's a two-month fetus, floating in amniotic fluid full of crack and alcohol? Not our problem. Her obesity makes her postoperative risk very high? We can't deny care on the basis of aesthetics.

There is tremendous hunger in our society for all of us to be seen as unique and precious individuals; yet there is an equal fear that we will be scorned or denied proper care on the basis of our attributes. For reasons of law, political correctness, and self-delusion, health care providers can't honestly admit our biases and judgments, which would at least permit us to face ourselves and our patients openly. So we all just keep it quiet and do things to patients we barely know for reasons that escape us.

Add to this the crush of time, financial pressures, the volume of patients we see, and the multitudinous demands pulling from a hundred directions, and the fact is that most health care workers know precious little about their patients. I can tell you her blood pressure this morning, her weight day by day, a list of all of her medical problems, and the sensitivity of her bacteria to twenty different antibiotics. But odds are I haven't a clue what she was doing the day before she got sick, or how she feels about her life.

Health care providers and families often miss the assumption that lurks at the core of the notions of autonomy, consent (guidance), beneficence, and nonmaleficence: all must be based on the *patient's* values, not those of the society, the family, or the provider. To carry out these ideas we must know the patient's values. This is not an encyclopedic task: we're not asking how the patient feels about everything under the sun. What we do need to be asking, however, is how the patient feels about items relevant to his illness and his treatments. The Advance Directive explicitly states that one reason for not providing life-sustaining treatment is if the burden of the therapy outweighs the likely benefits. But how much weight does the patient give to nausea, debility, fear, or grief? Does he worry more about his appearance or emotional or physical pain? Does she care about the demands she'll place on her family or the quality of her life before and after the illness or interventions? If we don't know these answers, we don't know much of anything.

The Context of the Individual

These later questions move toward a context we often miss in hospital care: Our tumultuous, urgent, amazingly costly, exciting time with a patient comprises a few moments out of a long lifetime. We see a few stressed interactions with a few of the people who have filled her life. We encounter her totally out of her environment, her clothes, her smells and home cooking and natural habits. Working from this terribly limited view of who the patient is, in all his or her dimensions of persona, will and spirit, we claim to know what's best for this infinite being under our care.

Up until 1970, the "patriarchal" model of medical decision-making looked like Figure 15.1. Our current, patient-centered ethics looks like Figure 15.2. Yet our practice of caring for a sick patient takes the form shown in Figure 15.3. The reality of the decision process looks much more like Figure 15.4, and the illness like Figure 15.5.

Our patient didn't live her life for the climactic moment when she could be rushed into the hospital, judged compliant or

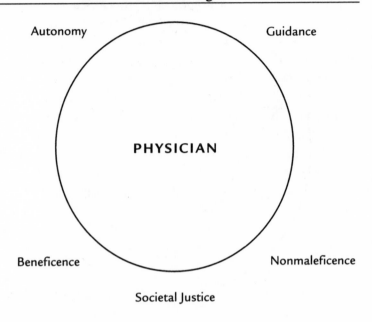

FIGURE 15.1 The "Patriarchal" Model of
Medical Decision-making

Autonomy   Guidance

PHYSICIAN

Beneficence   Nonmaleficence

Societal Justice

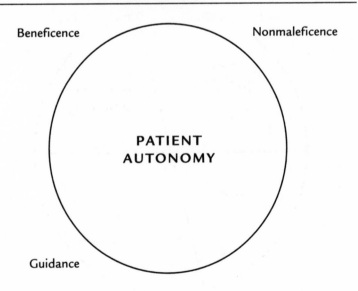

FIGURE 15.2 The Current American Notion of
Patient-centered Ethics

Beneficence   Nonmaleficence

**PATIENT
AUTONOMY**

Guidance

FIGURE 15.3 Our Practice of Caring for a Sick Patient

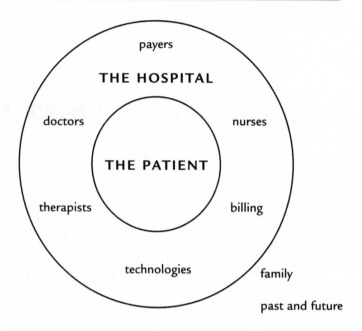

payers

THE HOSPITAL

doctors

nurses

THE PATIENT

therapists

billing

technologies

family

past and future

FIGURE 15.4 The Reality of the Decision Process

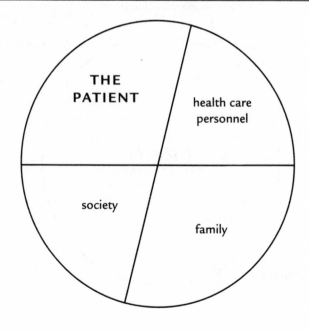

THE PATIENT

health care personnel

society

family

FIGURE 15.5 The Reality of the Illness

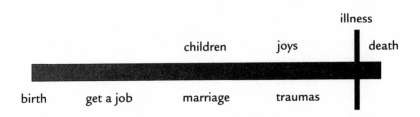

noncompliant, saved or not, and moved out to make room for the next "client." Rather, we are a short test, a trial by fire that will constitute just one of many passages in a long journey.

When we move our health care system out of the center of the picture, and a life's evolution to the center, the story reads so differently. Two such tales come to mind.

In *The Jewish Way in Death and Mourning*, Maurice Lamm recounted a parable of two sons in the womb. One is a skeptic, one a believer. They argue over what awaits them when they "die" out of the womb. The faithful son anticipates a "new great world" where they will eat through their mouths, hear through the ears on the sides of their heads, see great distances, and have their heads "up and free rather than down and boxed in."

The skeptical son sees all this as "an elaborate defense mechanism, a historically-conditioned subterfuge." He's certain they will simply "go with a bang. Our world will collapse and we will sink into oblivion. No more. Nothing. Black void."

> Suddenly the water inside the womb bursts. The womb convulses. Upheaval. Turmoil. Writhing. Everything lets loose. Then a mysterious pounding—a crushing, staccato pounding. Faster, faster, lower, lower.
>
> The believing brother exits. Tearing himself from the womb, he falls outward. The second brother shrieks—startled by the "accident"

befallen his brother. He bewails and bemoans the tragedy—the death of a perfectly fine fellow. Why? Why? Why didn't he take better care? Why did he fall into that terrible abyss?

As he thus laments, he hears a head-splitting cry, and a great tumult from the black abyss, and he trembles: "Oh my! What a horrible end! As I predicted!"

Meanwhile as the skeptic brother mourns, his "dead" brother has been born into the "new" world. The head-splitting cry is a sign of health and vigor, and the tumult is really a chorus of *mazel tovs* sounded by the waiting family thanking God for the birth of a healthy son.

Carl Sagan considers the images in near-death experiences—the turmoil, the release, the bright glowing light at the end of a tunnel, well-known family and friends waiting to receive the person who is dying. He suggests these are nothing more than remembrance of a vaginal birth. Perhaps, in his view, this is why so many physicists favor the "big bang" theory of the birth of the universe. Only those delivered by caesarian section could conceive of a "stasis" model for the cosmos's beginning.

For me, the pounding, crushing, and the howling secular dread of nothingness beyond sound awfully familiar. I participate in them several times a month. It's called cardiopulmonary resuscitation, or CPR. A dozen of us stand around a bed, desperately trying to hold closed the passage by which our patient's soul is attempting to be delivered into the life that follows. If James Hillman is right and our soul knows not just the past but also what lies ahead, perhaps those physicists and near-death travelers have seen where we're going.

"Jack and the Beanstalk" is a young man's tale, having to do with magic, leaving the mother, and meeting the terrifying, remote father. As so often, there's a treasure to be gained. Jack is sent to sell the family cow in a last desperate attempt to sustain a family whittled down to an impoverished mother and her son. He comes upon a little old man at the roadside (always in fairy tales such figures symbolize the connection with the ancients, the earth, the magically profound). They trade the cow for a handful of magic beans, and the boy marches home proud of his good fortune.

The mother, enraged, throws the beans out the window and ejects her stupid son from the house. Robert Bly here has suggested that the modern mother would solicitously support her son's self-esteem, cooing, "Why, how lovely! Let's put these beans on the mantel and we'll talk about them later," and with that the son's development, the adventure, the magic would all slam closed.

Though this tale is usually taken as a children's story, the previous Jewish parable draws the parallel between birth into this life and death into the next. As we approach death, we have the potential to go through an explosion of danger and transformation, understanding and resolution. Initiations bristle with pain, loss, and terrifying creation.

If we look openly and clearly at the participants in the end-of-life drama, we begin to see how unique each individual is and how powerfully that individuality alters the developments ahead. Is our patient a "believer" or a "skeptic"? Does he approach death with fear and hopelessness? Then perhaps we need to offer some insights that would help him see the process as one of growth, learning, and completion. Does the depth of her belief remove her from connection to those still around her in this life? Perhaps we could draw her vision back into this world long enough to complete the tasks she can still undertake for those she's loved.

And we all have roles in the "Jack and the Beanstalk" story. Health care providers are the mother who can smother our patients and families by emphasizing their debility and dependency or isolate them by throwing their essence, their unique histories and potentials, out the window while they yet live. We can encourage them and guide their adventure toward a place we cannot go, or we can make them dependent on us, trap them by the hearth, keeping everything focused on our own technology and plans.

These stories move the illness, the decay, even the death into the mythic positions usually occupied by dragons and giants. Today's health care worker could have been yesterday's rabbi or wizard. At our best, we could aspire to be the little old man at the side of the road who offers the magic beans.

As emphasized by Stephen Levine in *A Year to Live*, amazing growth, learning, and resolution often occur in the few days to months following a fatal diagnosis. Rapprochements, forgiveness, and love withheld for decades may burst forth as time runs out. It is the illness that rang the bell, that awakened the sleeping spirits: the members of Sleeping Beauty's court rise from their hundred-year slumber, gather around, and wait anxiously to hear what gift was spawned by the terrible curse. Whether or not we contain the illness and delay the death, we still have the opportunity to respond to the bell that tolled its message: "All has changed. Sleep no more. Time is short. You have a year to live—now what will you do with it?"

The answers to these questions can be pursued only if we first explore what is unique in this person. Jan Bernard and Miriam Schneider adapt five principals of spirituality from Father Santan Pinto. Of these, the fifth is: "'*God creates us as unique individuals.*' We each need to know as we journey toward death how precious and irreplaceable we are: our body, soul, and spirit are distinct expressions of the creative energy of the universe. This idea confers great value to each who dies. It allows us to accept gifts of the spirit graciously because we know we are important. It means we deserve to be among family and at home—in whatever sense of the word is appropriate—when we die. This principle also confers the great responsibility to seek out and honor each life, even those it may be more convenient to ignore."

Tasks

Some of what the individual may need to do is as remarkably straightforward as it is neglected. Wills and testaments. Is the wife's name on the bank account? Does the husband have a clue where the ketchup resides, or how to make a sandwich? Who gets the house? And how is everybody going to feel about that? How does one get a burial plot? Who's going to change the oil in the car?

I was riding through Manhattan with my dear friend Bobbi's parents in the front seat. Her mother was dying of cervical cancer. Her father turned to his wife and asked, "Marcia, where is your funeral plot?" I nearly exploded at his crassness. A little later she turned to him and fretted, "Hy, how are you going to take care of yourself? I think we need to find a good woman to take care of you when I'm not here." Only years later did I realize that they were doing the good work of caring for each other now, in the present, while they could.

Some tasks are a bit deeper. What are you going to regret not having said or done? Is there a question about life, about the world, about a loved one, that you never dared to ask? Ask it now. Don't be afraid. What are we going to do, kill you if we don't like your question?

And the deepest explorations, those of guilt and transcendence, of heaven and hell, judgment and forgiveness, move into the realm of faith and the eternal. I'll touch on this adventure more in a later chapter. Sadly, religion doesn't always seem to work to the benefit of the soul. "We're Christians, so we must do everything to stay alive." "It's a sin to give up." "We'll never forgive ourselves if we don't do everything to keep him alive." It is at such moments that the failure of faiths and health care systems to speak to one another is most glaringly obvious. We are at war; we don't share even a vaguely common language; and we refuse to hire translators. Chronic life support is mistaken for eternal life. Accepting death is equated with suicide or inadequate respect for life.

The Shadow

Here we move into the part of the individual or ourselves that we don't want to see, acknowledge, or face. It's what Carl Jung termed "the shadow," or another mythology called Ereshkigal, queen of the underworld. Though interpreted differently by different writers, the shadow is the sum of all the parts we were told were unacceptable, "bad," immoral, ugly, inadequate, despicable. It's what Luke Skywalker faces when he slays his "father" deep in the forest of Dagoba, only to discover his own face behind the mask.

Shadow may be "light" or "dark," valuable or harmful. But in either case, because we deny and suppress it, it manifests itself in our outer life in a twisted, chaotic way.

In the depths of a terrifying depression, I once asked a therapist, "What is this 'empty' place inside me, the one I work so hard and race around so much trying to 'fix' or avoid? It feels like a 'black hole' that would engulf me if I ever get too near it." George smiled and said, "Well, in Eastern philosophies, I believe that's where they'd expect to find God." There is a very strong sense that the shadow, that black, terrifying sum of all we've been told we must never on penalty of death admit is part of us, contains our greatest gifts, the key to our healing, the gems that most make us unique and of special value in this world.

And I suspect that the shadow is also why so many of us "marry our worst nightmare." Often we seek in another the parts we've denied in ourselves. The cold, fearful man finds a woman who is loving, emotional, and vital. The abuser finds a martyr. The giver finds one who needs. The woman who desperately seeks the family she never had finds a man who comes from and wants a big family, but in the end she is overwhelmed by it. The man whose sexuality is locked away in judgment seeks a woman who will draw it forth, then condemns her for her appetites.

Beyond the outer marriage of a "match made in heaven," we have also married our shadow, manifested in our vision of our mate. But then we gradually discover that we're profoundly uncomfortable with the differences between what we are and whom we've joined. We sought in the other the parts of ourselves we locked away. We locked them away because we were taught that they were unacceptable, perverted, bad. Now here we are with the person we hoped would unlock those qualities, bring them back into light. But for the

same reason we were taught to find those qualities despicable in ourselves, we soon find them to be so in our mate.

In a more Jungian sense, we internally marry our worst nightmare
when we accept and honor those qualities of ourselves that we had
stuffed in our bag of shadow.

Our society denies the darkness, the shadow, the "imperfect." And
like any deeply true thing, our denial only increases its power and
its demand to be acknowledged. If we believe only in goodness and
light, we will encounter evil and sin. If we deny the fire in our adolescents' bellies, they'll burn down the cities. If we make sex bad, our
radios and televisions will be happy to make idols of sexuality. The
day our technologic hubris denied death was the day our lives began dying.

The reason I mention shadow here is that a great deal of what
happens around the last of life is shadow work. If death is the ultimate failure, the bogeyman, the blackness reaching up from inside
every one of our cells to grab us, then when we move into death's
domain all other aspects of shadow scramble to be heard, now, while
there's still time.

The very sense of darkness has emotional, social, and historical
meaning. To Europeans for two thousand years, the darkness of
Africa and people of color was foreboding, unknowable, diabolical.
Medieval paintings showed the world with Abel's Europe white, at
the top; deceptive, sneaky Ham's Asia toward the bottom, or hell;
and Cain's black Africa on the west, the side of death. White Europeans projected much of their fear of their own shadow onto the
"Dark Continent" of Africa. When Joseph Conrad's Marlowe re-
coiled from "the horror, the horror" in *Heart of Darkness,* it was not
the Africans he had finally seen but the dark, twisted aspects of the
European tribe of which he was a part. On the other side of the looking glass, black Americans know all too well the feeling of being
"other," unwelcome, not equal. Many fear what treatment they will
receive at the hands of institutions they do not control.

So what shall we do with the shadow that grabs its last chance to be brought into the light of our consciousness and our daily lives? The man who was always a vigorous overachiever might yield to the depression that has stalked him his entire life. The wife who depended on him begins to prepare for self-sufficiency. Loving families may admit their resentments over whom was best loved and who best loves Mom, who wants to save her from death, who from suffering. We say, "Dad wouldn't want this," when what we really mean is, "I wouldn't"—or "I want Dad to be the kind of person who wouldn't accept such treatment."

Most of us have spent our lives keeping our shadow and our family's shadow stuffed away in an ever-expanding bag we drag around behind us. When our arms grow weary and our broken-field running lags, then the shadow starts leaking into the light. It's terrifying; it's startling; it's painful to face it in ourselves and our loved ones. But it's also a profoundly rich part of ourselves and one that the approach of death invites us to welcome home. In Gabriel García Márquez's *One Hundred Years of Solitude*, the eldest son appears after a long absence in a small Central American village. He is covered with tattoos and brings with him a strange, wild woman the villagers cannot understand. But he also brings the vitality, worldly wisdom, and daring that the dying community so desperately needs. And for this they kill him. This is the same way we tend to respond when the soul, long hidden, raises its head.

A Patient Case

I want to follow one patient through these last four chapters about various aspects of the soul. I ask you to consider what was healing and what wounding about the course he followed and what we did to him. Have you had similar experiences? What would you do differently, now, tomorrow, if you could?

~

Jay was a fifty-five-year-old truck driver who had continued to work through twenty-five years of diabetes. He'd raised two children and left or been left by two wives. When the going got rough, he moved to Redding so his daughter, Angie, could do what she'd sworn never to do—take care of him through his illness and eventual death.

During most of the time I cared for him, he seemed vigorous, virile, and independent. When presented with the prospect of kidney failure, he immediately chose peritoneal dialysis as the least likely to affect his life. After all the denying or being angry at his diabetes, he wasn't about to give it the satisfaction of limiting his lifestyle.

He subsequently suffered many of the ravages of diabetes: heart attacks, cardiac catheterization and coronary bypass, pneumonia, failing vision. Paralysis of some eye muscles ended his driving. He underwent multiple surgeries for clotted dialysis accesses and in his last four months was hospitalized five times for vomiting, dehydration, and heart failure. His last admission was for vertigo due to a stroke.

Three times I saw him become very discouraged and irritable. The first was when his heart trouble lasted for weeks in the hospital, possibly without the option of surgical treatment. The second came when he found that he was not a candidate for a transplant. Finally, the stroke brought him down. "I could handle it," he said, "but when will the next thing go wrong? Why keep fighting when there will always be another blow?"

After his death, his daughter Angie told me more about this man who had been my patient for three years. In Jay's childhood, he and his mother had been battered by his father, who was a rageful, bitter man. Unbeknownst to Jay, his mother gave up one child to adoption when his father ran off; by the time Jay was eighteen, she'd had to put her remaining son in a detention home. He never forgave her or women in general. She'd not protected him from his father, and now she'd abandoned him to the hard world.

His children were raised by a wife descending into alcoholism, and by Jay, who constantly battered them with rejection and anger. "Be a man; don't cry." "You're all to blame for my being upset. Now get out of my way!" His life had been one long battle for control—control over his emotions, over other people, over a world he couldn't trust. All he achieved was to push everyone away and drag his son into the same eons-old battle.

The domestic violence that had characterized his youth passed through him like the twisting helix of DNA. By the time his children left home, one to an early marriage, the other to a life of drugs, all they felt for him was fear. The love was gone.

Whenever people didn't do what they said or he wanted, he took it as a personal slap at him. Twelve years before, when his second marriage fell apart, it brought up all of his beliefs that everyone was out to get him. He went roaming from truck stop to truck stop in a murderous rage. One night a trucker heard his rampage and started talking to him about God. In 1985 Jay was "born again." Though he felt for the first time that "somebody was helping, that I didn't have to carry it all alone," the angers and resentments didn't change much. Still, knowing that he never would have the ultimate power gave him some feeling of release.

Over the subsequent years, he reestablished contact with his first wife and "adopted" eight surrogate grandchildren, who adored him as his own children could not.

He dealt with his diabetes by adamant denial, liberally sprinkled with waves of seething resentment. By the time the first organ failures from his diabetes began, he considered them a "wake-up call": "Listen, sucker, you didn't pay attention. All your anger and frustration didn't save you from your fate."

And now this damned illness had taken over his body, his spirit, and his dreams. The lifelong quest for control had been lost.

SIXTEEN

The Soul as Eternal Being: What I Came Here to Learn

They had been with me for "eternities," they said. I didn't fully understand this; I had a difficult time comprehending the concept of eternity, let alone eternities. Eternity to me had always been in the future, but these beings said they had been with me for eternities in the past. This was more difficult to comprehend. Then I began to see images in my mind of a time long ago, of an existence before my life on earth, of my relationship with these men "before." As these scenes unfolded in my mind I knew that we had indeed known each other for "eternities." I became excited. The fact of a pre-earth life crystallized in my mind, and I saw that death was actually a "rebirth" into a greater life that stretched forward and backward through time.

—Betty J. Eadie, *Embraced by the Light*

The Great Escape

When a patient dies, there is a small, trembling part of me that sighs in deep relief. As I confessed earlier, it comes from the part of me that knows we all make mistakes, often unnoticed, but that I'm expected never to make them. It's the part that fears my IV line may have become infected, my peritoneal catheter will perforate the intestine, the medicine I prescribed would eventually have killed the patient, or the lab test I didn't think of was the one that would have made all the difference.

As I leave the hospital bed now empty but for a body, this crummy part of me is reassured that anything I did wrong soon will be beyond discovery.

At least, in this world.

It's the opposite of Shakespeare's "The evil a man does lives after him; the good is oft interred with his bones" (*Julius Caesar*, Act III, Scene 2). In our culture's focus on the temporal body as the only life, the end of a life is the end of hope—but also the end of suffering and the wiping out of all the body's wounds, including those inflicted by people who meant to provide healing but achieved the opposite.

But is it so?

Much of modern end-of-life care is predicated on this belief. It becomes most clear in the contrast between "informed consent" and CPR that is automatically performed unless the patient has ordered otherwise. If I walked into your room, spoke not a word, rolled you off to surgery, and whipped out your gallbladder without your permission, I'd be in court before I could get my mask off. The charges would be assault and battery, denial of your autonomy, unwanted touching. If the procedure to which I exposed you had a 2 percent chance of working and a 12 to 20 percent chance of harming you, there would probably be twenty salivating lawyers outside the recovery room offering to sue me on your behalf.

In all of medicine, there is only one procedure that we routinely perform without informed consent: cardiopulmonary resuscitation. I don't know what we think we're doing to the rest of the organs and the spirit, but at least we resuscitate the lungs and heart. Why is CPR different from everything else we do? First, because of the presumption that everyone would want "everything" done. Second, because the Hippocratic (some say Hypocritic) oath says we should act first (but not only) to guard life.

The Advance Directive and Right to Die movements challenge the first presumption. Regarding the second, most physicians are unaware of the "not only" part, or that the oath's commandment that we ease suffering often requires us to permit death to proceed. The snake that entwines the caduceus, the symbol of my profession, is not just the messenger of Apollo, a god long departed. It's also the symbol of the cycle of life and death, of transformation, of shedding the old to reveal the newly reborn. Yet contemporary medicine acts as if we have a sacred responsibility to prevent death at all costs.

At the base of it, I believe we use a sort of inversion of Pascal's wager, which I'll describe later in this chapter. If we do CPR and win, even in 2 percent of cases, we're heroes. If we lose, our perception is either that the dead body will not suffer from our assault, or that at least "dead men tell no tales."

But is it so?

When I was at El Camino Hospital in Mountain View, California, several years ago, we held a conference about the ICU experience. Four survivors of months-long ICU stays were invited back, with their families, to tell us what it was like. Three hundred doctors, nurses, therapists, and administrators gathered in the audience to receive their applause for our brilliance and our commitment to these beloved souls.

In their different ways, three of four began, "I will never forgive you for keeping me alive. The rest of my wrecked life I will carry the memory of all I and my family suffered at your hands. It wasn't worth it."

Gulp.

The usual response of physicians to such a story is, "Ungrateful wretches! Depressed whiners! Get over it!"

In their way, I believe these patients were trying to say that the cure had created its own illnesses, that those wounds lived on, and that their persistence in every moment, every thought, felt far worse than a peaceful or even a painful death. Had we let that ending come to pass, they would not have suffered, at least not in this particular way. The experience of heroic intervention had welded these patients to their experience of suffering.

But is it so?

Is There an Eternal Soul?

In brief, I can't scientifically prove it, one way or the other. I suspect this is the least scientifically testable of any of the aspects of "soul." This is the leap of faith that separates the "believer" from the "skeptic" son in the Jewish parable related in Chapter 15. It is the leap of faith that carries Indiana Jones to the Holy Grail, that separates scientific materialism from mystic unification. Back when the original monastic hospices evolved into hospitals, science smote religion a mighty blow. Then and there, our material bodies became separated from everything else in the universe.

Can we know? In scientific terms, that is, hypotheses verifiable by physical signs, it's pretty rough. Most of our "experience" of the eternal comes from sensations belonging more to the "legacy" or the "*one*." A child is visited in a dream by a dead parent. My friend Clarence experiences his son's death in a car accident very differently from what he'd been told had happened; later, it turns out the events unfolded exactly as he'd seen them. An angel deflects us from the path of the onrushing truck, or voices speak to us in dreams or reverie.

The dear departed's legacy lives on, whatever the mechanism. So many of us have visceral reactions when we see a road-kill rabbit or a forest clear-cut. When we come upon a silted-over salmon spawning area, perhaps we are reminded of parts of ourselves that never saw the light. And there are deeper reactions: an old woman dying alone and unmourned reminds us of our own tenuous connection to those around us. Even the cool isolation of scientific reason can't fool us that we're not part of these beings, and they not *one* with us. Even the certainty that infuses a congregation of believers may speak more of the joy of the *one* than the embrace of the one God.

Can we glimpse the eternal? Near-death experiences describe a glorious calm, illumination, a release and eventual return to those we love and by whom we have always been loved. But is that reality seen through the eyes of our eternal being? Or is it merely a memory of a vaginal birth, as Carl Sagan and others have suggested? Is our brain desperately scrambling for more endorphins as it dies, trying to protect us from the terror and horror of disintegration?

Some religions go to great lengths to describe the afterlife, which generally offers what was least attainable in this life. The Koran of Islam, struggling its way thirstily out of the desert, opens with a wondrous description of the Garden where water flows eternally and beautiful maidens bring endless bounties of food and drink. The Bible and Torah describe a blissful afterlife of harmony and peace very unlike our tumultuous, uncertain world. Are these tales just the efforts of organized religions to act as the "opiate of the masses," or is the situation the reverse: that science has anesthetized our consciousness to the true visions of the soul? Buddhism as ever takes a third path. Since this life is only illusion, the afterlife is the only genuine life, no longer blinded by sensory overload.

Now, that certainly takes the sting out of insurance companies' refusal to approve treatments, doesn't it?

Can we experience the soul directly? There are individual experiences of the departing spirit, usually by those who have worked closely and openly with the dying and tuned themselves to what inhabits the mystery and the darkness. Miriam Schneider described one such experience in *The True Work of Dying* (with Jan Bernard):

> I am not sure when in my nursing career I became consciously aware that something or someone fills the room of the dying one. It is a profound presence. This awareness began to intensify after I attended several deaths. Initially, I began to recognize a change in the atmosphere upon entering the room of someone close to death. I had grown accustomed to the emotional and physical changes a person undergoes shortly before death. The spiritual changes were more subtle. I gradually recognized as I became quieter within my heart that the spiritual growth of someone close to death was obvious. In time I

could simply walk past a room and sense these changes and how a body was close to death without directly perceiving the dying one's physical or emotional changes.

… Just as I was remembering Steve's passage, I felt someone kiss me on the top of my head and a voice saying thank you and good-bye. I looked around somewhat startled. I thought I had been quite alone. Indeed, as I looked around, I saw nothing but an empty room.

What was this presence that filled the room and kissed her in passing? Was it the scent of cells dying? Was it the subliminal rhythm of a body breathing out more than it was breathing in? Was it her own intuition and devotion revealing itself? Or was it the manifestation of an eternal soul?

Jelaluddin Rumi, the wondrous poet and dervish, describes a bit of life in *These Branching Moments:* "We talk about this and that. There's no rest/except on these branching moments."

What we do today is ride out but a few moments branching to we know not what, wrapped in the two wings of a vast eternity. But is this only poetry, just so many shimmering words? To what organ and from what organ in us do such words speak? Are they hallucinations? A swamp of overheated endorphins? We don't yet have the PET (positron emission tomography) scanner that can differentiate an experience of what is external (in scientific terms, "real") from that which is generated by memory or spirit (in spiritual terms, "real," in scientific terms, "bogus" because not physically verifiable).

In the Acknowledgments I mentioned Dr. Beatrice Tucker, who ran the Maternity Center for home obstetrics in Chicago. A few months ago, a young man at a workshop offered me a dream he'd had the night before. In less than two days, he'd already figured out I was a loser. He was kind enough to tell the group, "I really appreciate Bruce's being here because he's shown me that if I don't do my work, I could end up like him when I get old." So you can imagine how much I looked forward to hearing his pithy nocturnal revelation.

He described seeing me as I was dressed that day, in scrub suit and jogging shorts, walking toward him down a long, antiseptic hallway that was most likely in a hospital. Behind me hurried a hundred "disembodied spirits" (sort of like ghosts or ghouls), reaching toward me. All they wanted was for me to feel their pain—not cure it, not be devoured by it, not fix it, not be tied to it—just feel it for a moment and they would be all right. But instead I turned away.

I've never heard a more accurate description of how I and, I suspect, many other health care providers feel when our patients deluge us with their needs, demands, and hopes. We derive a great sense of status and self-worth from helping others. But there's the constant terror that we'll be overwhelmed, disappear into the endless swamp of hunger, the expanding wounds, the impossibility of cure.

Later that day, I asked him to describe the "disembodied spirits." He remembered only one, a tall, scrawny old lady in a pixie haircut and loads of jewelry. The funny thing was that when she talked, her dentures clattered. It was dear Beatrice, I have no doubt.

He'd known me less than a day. I'd never talked of Tux, yet here she was in his dream, speaking to me thirty years later. Her coyote magic was as alive as ever. Now, how are you going to explain that with endorphins?

Brian Weiss, the academic psychiatrist mentioned in Chapter 14, "The Soul's Calling," described in three books his gradual conversion to a belief in past and future lives. He took his clients through hypnosis back to the times of the traumas that caused present-tense problems. Suddenly one or another was describing scenes from past lives. All right, that's a nice metaphor. But then other voices arose, the "masters." They began referring to facts in Weiss's life that only he could have known. And eventually two or more clients would precisely describe events they'd shared in past lives.

Because he so carefully monitored and described his gradually crumbling skepticism, Weiss convinced me as well. I suspect the mystics and gurus, seers and shamans, priests and rabbis and muftis all saw very well what we of science have learned to deny. There is something that lives on, that remembers, that can return still wounded but determined to heal from other lifetimes.

And if all of that doesn't ring your bell, settle for Pascal's wager. The question posed to Pascal, a seventeenth-century philosopher and mathematician, was, Is there a God? His answer was, Say yes. If there isn't, you've lost nothing. If there is and you guess wrong, you may just have lost everything for all eternity.

In the arena of medical thanatology (the "science" of death and dying), I'd put the wager this way: Is there an eternal soul on which we leave the marks of our transgressions and the glow of our love? Better answer yes. If we're wrong, nothing has been lost. If we're right but we treated the living person as if her body and essence were just a bit of refuse to be discarded when the last breath passed away, we're all in big, big trouble.

How Shall We Treat this Eternal Soul?

Looked at that way, the idea that we can flail away at a critically ill body as if death will erase any errors we make may not be the best wager after all. In fact, it may be the worst. Compassion, tenderness, and heedful listening might have had a far greater healing effect on the departing soul than ignoring its wishes, cracking its body's chest, ramming tubes into its bodily orifices, and driving its family from the room where its body was trapped in its final moments.

So let's say there is an eternal soul. Decisions around illness and the end of life now look like Figure 16.1. The illness in context looks like Figure 16.2. What did it come here to do, and what are our responsibilities to it as it passes through?

What Is the Eternal Soul Here to Do?

Leaving aside secular materialism, which sees the soul as an aberrant endorphin assault on the rational neuronal net of dopaminergic nerve endings, most religious and philosophical traditions see this lifetime as a test of some sort. Maybe it's something like an eternal forest sprung wondrously from new seeds, or a trial by fire. Often

FIGURE 16.1 Decisions Around Illness and the End of Life

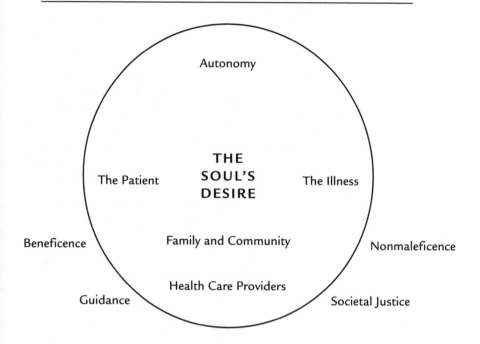

Autonomy

The Patient

THE SOUL'S DESIRE

The Illness

Beneficence

Family and Community

Nonmaleficence

Health Care Providers

Guidance

Societal Justice

FIGURE 16.2 The Illness in Context

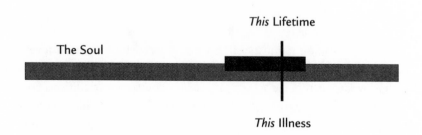

This Lifetime

The Soul

This Illness

life seems to be a long, long class with incomprehensible lessons taught in a foreign tongue. The soul must see it as a deeply perplexing, often amusing meander. For many, it's nothing but a dream.

If we believe that we live this life to *earn*, by moral rectitude and good deeds, a pass to heaven, then what does illness offer? For the patient, it's a chance to go through this trauma well, to honor the spirit and act in such a way toward those around him that he will bring himself and them closer to God and healing. He should seek and offer forgiveness. Patient, family, and caregivers should all attempt to correct the wounds our professional and personal errors have caused in the past. We should prove ourselves worthy.

This view would command the caregiver to support to the very last the patient's ability to act, to manifest, to touch. We should draw the dialogue toward what is unsettled, unresolved, bitter. We must reach into the place that is aching, needing attention. The god who wounds is the god who cures. The wound is the blessing, the opening, the way. Christ consciousness is not confined to Christians; perhaps we each need to be the way and the salvation of those we love. The purpose of our medicines should be to calm pain enough to maximize function, not to numb existential pain.

Existential pain? What in the world is that? It's the grief at all our life could have achieved but did not, all our soul intended to do but did not. Suddenly confronted with a clock running out, we ache that our lives could have been otherwise. If we numb the pain, we die in a narcotic peace. If we do not, we may change our fate.

There is a puritanical, judgmental streak in many health care professionals who resist "overmedicating" a patient. It is indeed a fine line, trying not to occlude or impair consciousness any more than necessary while keeping physical pain at a "tolerable" (to whom?) level. Each patient must tell his caregivers which "pain" hurts most—physical pain, the existential pain of not being able to complete what she'd come here to do, fear, debility, uncertainty. One Hospice volunteer recounted the death of her sixteen-year-old son: "He wanted so much to be present, to feel everything that was happening at the end. So for him, unlike most of my patients, 'comfort measures' that clouded his alertness were profoundly uncomfortable." For others, the awareness of discomfort may be more terrifying than being medicated into coma.

If we believe that our soul came here to *learn* and undergo certain emotional or physical experiences it can carry back to the spiritual realm, then what does illness offer? It can teach us what is left after we have accepted loss and pain. Illness can strip away the external trappings of our lives, cutting us down to the essence of what we really are or what really matters. We find the power in powerlessness, the depth of connection and caring between ourselves and others, and our profound ability to touch and shape them as they shape us in our moment of vulnerability. The approach of death certainly gives us the opportunity to experience the intensity of our emotions—rage, sadness, grief, love, hope, despair, enlightenment. The pain of the body. The pain of shame and doubt. The aching of the spirit in its lifelong isolation. The grief over what seems unattainable.

Here, the caregiver could look deeply into the patient's eyes and find what she's seeking. What does she seem to be holding on to? What experience was needed but hasn't yet happened? What did she always need to do but never quite got to? What does she need to feel, just once or just once more, before she dies?

I can visualize my patient's body, like something in a bizarre Hieronymus Bosch painting, strapped to the bed, immobilized, moldering. A desperate little red spirit is trapped inside pounding at its cage of ribs. The body has become the sum of all the dis-eases of illness, the painful nausea and loss of function, the humiliations of incontinence and smell and appearance. How can we assist the soul in escaping a body no longer suitable for manifesting love and joy?

Our Responsibilities to the Soul

Our end-of-life technology does indeed provide the soul with abundant experiences to carry on to the other side. And we are granted remarkable power to determine what those last experiences will be. Was the person's essence heard and cherished? Did we lift her beyond her mortal constraints, or were our hospital staff a thousand Lilliputians strapping her down? Did we treat our patients with respect or dismissal? Will the departing soul conclude from its final treatment that life is nothing but pain and endless woundings? Does every IV hurt and every treatment cause harm? Or will we demonstrate that every injury may provide an opportunity for healing and for love? I've seen the bodies of patients in persistent vegetative state (irreversible coma) tense up and stream tears when turned by one attendant, yet relax and radiate calmness, even happiness, when touched by another. One physician can speak and the whole room goes tense. Another enters, and even the flowers seem to open.

If the soul comes to learn from experience, then caregivers and family members can greatly affect what the learning is and how it is interpreted in these intense hours just before passing over to what follows this existence. Scott Peck particularly addressed this issue in *Denial of the Soul*. Euthanasia, he said, makes sense if we believe we end when we die. Then no pain, no suffering, no learning has any value, and we should just get it over with. He sees this perspective as a fundamental denial of the soul. If instead we see illness and death, even pain, as teachers to a consciousness that will live on, then premature anesthesia and euthanasia rip away all the opportunities for growth the illness made available. If we believe there is nothing to learn and no growth to occur, we learn nothing and shrivel away. Like the tree that doesn't fall in the forest if no one is there to hear it, perhaps even a soul disappears if we deny its existence long enough.

A thirty-nine-year-old man died at our hospital recently. He'd had lymphoma twenty years ago. He was now suffering the late consequences of the radiation that cured his tumor but had become its own disease. Most of his last four months were spent in the hospital. In the end, he wanted to die at home but wanted to be kept alive if possible. His wife wanted to wrap him in blankets and shelter him from the pain of dying. It crushed her that the last of his life was such a struggle. She wanted him home but was terrified of his dying there. Each had internally inconsistent desires.

In the "yes-or-no" mode of linear thought, we chose: he died in the hospital with her sitting by the wall as the nursing and medical staff warred about whether to give more morphine to ease his suffering or less so he could live longer.

In looking back, I read the tale this way: what they wanted was not so very far apart. He could have died at home, on a ventilator, wrapped in her love and with sufficient morphine to ease his suffering. What prevented it was her fear of his death and his unrealistic hope for continued life. What we failed to address were these fears and contradictions. His soul learned that he would die isolated from those who would have loved him, surrounded with conflict. Hers learned that she was powerless either to create the end she hoped to give him or to protect him. And we all, every one of us, learned just how horribly isolated and alone we were. It could have been otherwise.

A fifty-nine-year-old patient of mine had been depressed and isolated his whole life. He didn't like people close to him, felt very much alone and hopeless. He liked his messy, unkempt house just the way it was and didn't want anybody else in it. His diabetes had reached the point that he'd need dialysis to survive. The morning I walked in to place his dialysis line, the room was dark and silent, and he didn't move. At first I thought he was dead. When he finally did rouse himself, it was to tell me he didn't want dialysis, that his life was over and he was going to die.

At that point, I normally would have hurried out and written a "do not resuscitate order" or prescribed antidepressants. As it happened, I'd just come back from the seminar where I was told about that dream of a legion of patients demanding that I simply witness their pain. Perhaps I'd not turn away, just this once, to see how it went. So I sat down on his bed, held his hand, and said, "OK. We don't have to start dialysis. It's your choice. Now, is there anything you need to complete before you die so you'll feel you've done what you

need to?" He couldn't think of anything. Well, maybe he should contact his wife, who had divorced him twelve years before. And then
there was the son he'd left as an infant. And he needed to get a place
set up for his dog. And some writing he'd always hoped to do.

All of this was in the area of "legacy," but what struck me was the
man I found in his room the next morning. The blinds were drawn
back; he was energetic and determined and anxious for my visit. He'd
decided he'd need at least four months to do all this stuff, so would
we please start dialysis to give him this time? Through focusing on
what remained to be settled, he in fact discovered a buried part of
himself. He has become the life of the party at dialysis, joking with
the nurses and other patients, concerned for how they're doing. He's
a vibrant man with much to offer and thoroughly enjoying his experience of himself as this long-buried, newly discovered being.

His need didn't devour me but enlightened me. Watching his soul
manifest itself touched mine deeply and showed me a way to joy. An
illness such as a stroke or heart attack might not have left him the
chance for healing. But renal failure, with its chronic sick/well split
and dependence on daily interaction with others, suited his soul's
yearning perfectly.

And is this life just an *illusion*, a Kabuki show acted out this side
of a hung sheet? If so, what practices will guide us to real understanding? Meditation if you can do it. Dreams if you work at remembering them. Hypnosis, trance work, spiritual contemplation,
prayer. All the stuff that doesn't fit into the schedule or the payment
structure of a hospital. Jan Bernard and Miriam Schneider wrote,
"The physical dwelling we call home is really just a symbol of the
home we feel inside, but the physical space is important to us because we go home to be ourselves. It's the refuge from a world filled
with demands for our time, energy, and resources." To what extent
do we create a refuge, and to what extent do we just multiply a lifetime's barrage of distracting demands? If we caregivers could picture
ourselves as part of the illusion, one phrase in some particularly net-
tlesome riddle, much would change. We'd be less desperate to be

"right," to "win," and instead keep part of ourselves free to watch and learn. What did the room look like as we struggled and stumbled? What made me miss that diagnosis, put that line in too quickly, push for this or that decision? How are her eyes changing as I speak? Do I feel her drawing closer to or farther from me as the treatments proceed? Is she becoming closer to or farther from her family? Herself? What's happening to her spirit?

I once duked it out with a sixty-eight-pound Vietnamese lady who'd had open-heart surgery. I refused to send her home until she ate; she refused to eat until I sent her home. Her malnutrition and stubbornness were going to wipe out all the benefits we'd achieved with our very expensive and invasive cardiac surgery.

After ten days of this conflict I gave up and discharged her. So there! Three months later I ran into her at her son's car-repair business. She was still sixty-eight pounds but chipper as a fine bird and thoroughly in control of everything happening in the garage. She cackled at me from her perch cross-legged atop one of the cars and wolfed down chopsticks-full of rice with evident gusto. She and I both knew just then what only she had known in the hospital: her soul saw me as just a fleeting illusion; if she closed her eyes, I'd go away.

Illness and death become the gossamer ripplings through which we can discern the soul at work. If we let go of our attachments to fear and victory, to status and power, we discover just beneath the surface a vibrant being working toward something it has sought its entire life. A patient may have nothing left with which to convey this but a glance or a change in his breathing pattern, or a brief grasp of my hand, but that being is there, and but for my illusions I could experience this with him.

Acts. Approaching God. Forgiveness. Healing. Learning. Truly seeing. Being touched. These are the offerings of every illness and every death. It is the eternal soul that will carry these with it. It is its legacy that leaves them in the world with us.

I described Jay's "individual" soul qualities in the previous chapter. He chose to control his death much as he'd tried to control his life, but this time with a grace that had often eluded him. One morning on rounds, I discovered him curled up in a fetal position. He told me in a barely audible voice that he'd had enough of vomiting and pain and couldn't stand one more day of wondering what disaster would strike next.

When I turned on the light, he curled deeper into himself, as if expecting me to strike him. I bent down to look at his face. Finally he responded: "Give me some insulin so I can end this." Over my shoulder, Jack Kevorkian rattled his black cape. I could swear I heard half a dozen lawyers opening their valises by the door.

"I can't do it, Jay. It's illegal."

He nodded, knowing that would be the answer. "Then I want to stop dialysis. How long will that take?"

I answered that he, his family, the nurses, and I would have two or three long weeks ahead of us. That, he decided, was how it would be.

Angie concurred with his decision. He'd always wanted to have his way, and he'd come to hate the uncertainty of this life. Some part of her that had never asked for him to show up on her doorstep was relieved that the endless weekends spent away from her family at the hospital, the terror every time the phone rang after nine P.M.— What did he need now? Was he dead? Did she have to take him back to the emergency room (ER) in the middle of the night and still function tomorrow at work?—would come to an end. Unable to manage her family, her job, and her father's death at home, she decided to place him in a nursing home.

The next morning, a dozen children, grandchildren, and friends jumbled together in Jay's room. I thought perhaps he'd managed to die, and they were mourning. To my astonishment, my shell of a patient was sitting up holding court. He'd reverted to the vital, humorous man I remembered from the years before. "My God, Jay," I said, "you look great! Now what are we going to do?" He laughed and said we'd best get on with getting him placed. He was going to enjoy these last few days.

As I fumbled, trying to figure out what to do about this resurrection (surely not one of the lectures in medical school—doctors are the only ones who are supposed to resurrect people), my words addressed the family's questions—How would the end go? Would he suffer much? What if he changed his mind? What should they do during this period?

One "adopted" grandson, a twelve-year-old, turned to me and half whispered, "I just want you to tell him I'm really going to miss him." His grandfather was only four feet away, yet the two communicated through me as if I were the intercom between this world and a place to which his grandfather had already departed.

As the meeting concluded, Jay put his arm around me and said, "I know this is hard for you. Don't feel like you did anything wrong. In 1985, I was born again. That was great, but this is much better. I know I'll never have to have another needle in my arm, another test, never have anything done I don't want. It's the best gift I could have." The radiance that surrounded him buoyed everyone in the room.

Jay had come back into his power and his delight in life. Not one person in that room, even those beginning to miss him desperately, considered making any move to deter him from his choice.

What would Jay's soul carry from this illness and death that his life might not otherwise have shown him? Angie felt he'd always refused to accept help, to admit need. The illness had forced him to rely on others, even to treat others well so they'd help him. He'd learned he could be like that, and that people cared enough about him to respond.

After a huge, nearly physical fight with Jay three weeks before his death, Angie stomped out and didn't return his calls for two days. The gift to her: she realized that she was an adult now and he could never attack her again. And Jay, seeing his old, violent self, was deeply apologetic and horrified at who he'd been all those years. He saw the anger and the hurt it caused, and it left him.

For the first time in his life, he became peaceful. The grace that religion suggested finally became the stuff of his daily life. He "mended fences" with the many people he felt he'd harmed and forgave himself near the end. The day before his death, he smiled at Angie and his son, A.J., and said, "I'm almost there."

For all the children he'd taken in, all the battles and events, he concluded, "You don't know how many lives you've touched until it comes to this." He discovered he'd never be ruler of the universe, never be in control, and he felt better for it. He felt satisfied in himself.

He also found satisfaction with his world and his story. For the first time ever, he praised his mother for the hard choices she'd had to make and how hard she'd tried. He'd never thought of her as having a rough time, or of how it must have hurt to do what she'd had to in order to try to make good lives for her sons. Two weeks before Jay's death, the brother he didn't know he had found him and came to Redding for a visit. As the two brothers reviewed the adoption record, they discovered in their mother's words a depth of love and daring neither had believed was there.

Several times in his last days, Jay told visitors I was his best friend. I was so startled, I had to ask Angie what he meant. She told me he felt that he could truly trust, that he was truly seen and loved for who he was, and that he was protected in a way he'd never felt before. I don't know where he got all this feeling. I did very little; my time and energy weren't a thousandth of what Angie had devoted to this man who had been so hard on her. But this was one of the lessons his soul chose to take from the illness and death by which we all were raised up.

SEVENTEEN

The Soul as Legacy: Beneath the Stones, These Words

> *"My father's people say that at the birth of the sun and of his brother the moon, their mother died. So the sun gave to the earth her body from which was to spring all life, and he drew from her breasts the stars. The stars he threw into the night sky to remind him of her soul. So there's the Camerons' monument. My folks' too, I guess."*
>
> —James Fenimore Cooper,
> *The Last of the Mohicans*

JUST AS THIS WORLD leaves its last marks on the eternal soul, the departing soul is determined to leave behind something for those who shared its time here. This legacy occupies much of our ego's thoughts and deeds when time grows short.

We tend to envision legacy in terms of bank accounts and titles to property, objects we've collected and debts we've incurred. But the soul traffics in other currency.

What is it that our soul would hope to have live on? In the words of Stephen Levine, from *"Who Dies? An Investigation of Conscious Living and Conscious Dying,* Who dies? What survives? How does the clear, bright wind from each death revitalize this twisting flame of immortality?"* I believe that as our bodies contract until they are nothing but smoke, our lives are distilled into our greatest or most poignant gift: the stories by which we will be remembered.

A World of Stories

Many native societies construct the map of their environment out of songs and morality tales. In *The Songlines*, Bruce Chatwin described how the Aborigines of Australia understand their world. For native people in many lands, every curve, every rock, each tree in their world tells a particular story of great meaning to the people. Those of us whose ancestors arrived here more recently retain diluted and somewhat detached mementos of such stories when we visit "Lover's Leap," "Hellpass Lake," "Hoboken, New Jersey," or "Jim Taylor, Pennsylvania."

Nevertheless, though we seldom notice it, we too understand our world through the stories a place or a name brings to mind. "The King" lives on in Graceland at least as vividly and potently as he ever did in life. "The Duke" still models American political discourse and the notion of what a man should be.

I interned at Chicago Wesley Memorial Hospital. This was a gold coast institution so ritzy-ditzy, it still had the chutzpah to put the well-to-do on a special ward. Senile rich folks on intravenous nutrition were served steaming trays of steak and lobster they couldn't recognize as food, and only certain carefully selected house officers were allowed to attend such glamorous minor deities.

Rushing to work one crystal-clear dawn, I was startled to discover makeshift tents and altars lining the last three blocks of my walk from Michigan Avenue to the hospital. The queen of the Gypsies had just died at Wesley. I found myself suddenly transformed into a full-time altar boy in a Gypsy shrine; for several years thereafter, no self-respecting Gypsy would have thought of dying anywhere but Saint Wesley's. We now had a place on their map that had nothing to do with longitude and latitude. Our business office didn't have a clue how status and finances were measured in this parallel realm that occupied our same place in the universe.

The few stories modern Americans hear seem to be written in courts and tabloids or come pouring from the televisions that have replaced our interest in those nearest to us. Whose story of a trip to the grocery store could hope to compete with the latest TV cop show? Why listen to a cousin sing a lament of her broken heart when the Spice Girls can leap all over the place in a million-dollar video?

Who are these people with whom I've shared so much of my life? What matters most to them? What do their lives have to tell me about the human condition and about myself? Come to think of it, I don't know.

The prologue to one edition of *Tales of the Thousand and One Nights* described a childhood in Baghdad. When the sun set and the candles came on, neighbors turned to one another for entertainment. The best storyteller was not the one with the most words or the most resonant voice; it was the wily old lady most in touch with the rhythms of the night, the one who could sense her audience's yearnings and aches. Yearn they did, as we all do, for something to make sense of our lives; it was a fortunate neighborhood that had such a one to light the night.

What would it take to make us turn from the boob tube toward those around us, and from there inward to our own hearts? If we ever did pause to look around us, who would be ready to speak? What would they say about the lives we've shared? Who will help me find my authentic voice?

True Futility

Nowadays doctors are very concerned about "futile" care near the end of life. As discussed in Chapter 7, we apply this term to therapies that offer little or no benefit. But for every patient I see caught in the web of "futile" technologic care, I see a hundred whose last of life is made futile by our failure to make of their lives a story worth remembering. What is futile is not our technology but how we neglect the gifts, stifle the yearnings, of the last of life.

So what are the stories we could be creating for our patients, our loved ones, and ourselves? Let me tell you a few tales.

A Thousand and One Nights

The Woman Who Turned to Stone

Ernlé Young, a wonderful ethicist from Stanford University, tells the story of an eighty-six-year-old woman with "fifteen organ-system problems, at least six of which were potentially fatal." Through two harrowing months, her daughter and granddaughter sat twelve-hour shifts at her bedside. Their expectations were totally unrealistic; they were sure Jesus would heal the silent old woman because she'd had an audience with the pope, and the family battled her caregivers for control of her care.

It was clear she wasn't going to survive, and her care was therefore futile. Finally, an attending physician who was going off service met with the family and said, "I'm off duty, it doesn't affect me one way or the other, but I feel we're harming your mother without benefit. We're all caught in a power struggle. I'd ask you to use your love for her to think about what is most kind, rather than what you most want for yourselves."

They consented to stop life support, and she died. Then they got to fighting over the autopsy.

The story the family was writing was about a struggle to protect one they loved. It was a story with miraculous promises and legions of enemies. The setting was one of devotion patiently and unrelentingly demonstrated in the midst of a war.

The family may have felt that the moral of the story was that they fought an evil and unconcerned juggernaut that rolled over them nevertheless. Or that Jesus decided and they obeyed Him. Maybe the devil won this time, or was it that they did all they could, all that was in their power, and therefore Mother or Grandmother sits comfortably on the heavenly throne earned by the sum of her goodness and their devotion?

I would tell the story this way: twelve hours a day for sixty days, each of two family members cherished this woman enough to sit by her bed. They placed her meaning above all the demands of their usual lives. Tragically, they and everyone around them were trapped in Third Chakra, in power and control; all the stories of her life and death were held captive behind that battlefield of metal, plastic, and blood.

The 720 hours each of them spent with her had great meaning and immense potential for healing. What did we do with that time? What guidance did the caregivers offer to help those women make it precious and worthwhile?

This is a story told hundreds of times a day in every hospital, and it is one that could have been written by O. Henry: she cuts off her hair to buy him a chain for his beloved watch; he sells his watch to buy her a set of combs for her beautiful hair. We and the families struggle to the death with our entire hearts and souls to "save" our patients, yet when we look in the mirror we see enemies, prisoners, and victims. The patient dies and we all walk away defeated. The one thing we can all be certain will survive—our memories of this person and of the last of his or her life—was never attended to. It glowers forth from the grave like some disfigured monster.

He Was a Man Just Like You

A forty-three-year-old developmentally delayed man, functionally age six, was admitted with heart failure. With his aortic valve closing down, he could barely breathe. He'd passed out three times in the past three weeks from lack of blood supply to his brain.

The primary-care doctor and cardiologist told the family he should be "no code" since his quality of life didn't justify cardiac catheterization or surgery. When he went into frank heart failure, we rushed him to surgery and he died on the table.

The family perceived the events as reinforcing an entire lifetime of neglect; of being treated as less than others; of mockery, struggle, and hopelessness. His mother and two brothers, who loved him dearly and were torn apart by how he'd been seen as less than human, are even now trying to find a way to heal the wound caused by his once again being abandoned by those who were supposed to treat him with respect.

The moral of the story? From the medical standpoint, that the Americans with Disabilities Act threatens us with legal action if we consider disability in deciding to limit what resources we provide to a patient. He received appropriate care considering the fragility of his condition.

From the patient's standpoint, he enjoyed his food and his friends and was pretty much as happy and troubled as any six-year-old—and now he's dead.

From the family's viewpoint, this was one more wounding rather than a final honoring of this boy-man. It seems to show that the world still hasn't learned how to love those who don't fit the "norm." What began as a genetic condition at conception or birth became a wounding of the entire family by society. Like a break in the genetic code, this tragic story may cascade through generations to come.

Will You Forgive Me?

A sixty-year-old Costa Rican man was conscious but dying from dead bowel. Ten to twenty family members were in constant attendance. They fretted over the latest laboratory test results, his vital signs, his pain, and what one or another nurse said. We all knew he'd die within three days, and I'd told him this at the bedside with his family at his side.

The tension was rising. There was another frenzied crescendo of "Can't we do something?" He seemed to be receding into the crypt

even as his pulse beat on. I didn't know what to do. All of my con-
sultants had headed for the hills. Walking into that room was like
walking defenseless into a car crash.

For reasons I can't explain, I said to the entire family and the patient, "You know Manuel is dying. He knows it, as you all do. I want
each of you to think about what you'll regret not having said or done
before he dies. Is it that you need to tell him that you love him? Will
you feel bad if you don't embrace him, or he you? Are you still pissed
off that he took your bike away when you were thirteen? Whatever.
The greatest gifts you can exchange now are truth and peace. Please
do it quickly, while there's time."

Everyone froze, looking at me as if I'd spoken in a foreign tongue.
(Actually, it was Spanish, which they knew quite well.) Eventually
his wife leaned close and spoke softly to this man she'd loved most
of her life. "Can you ever forgive me?" she whispered.

His eyes snapped open for the first time since his failed surgery.
"Ay, no, *cara,* all these years I wondered if you'd ever forgive me!"
She hugged him and they cried, and it was as if the manacles that
had chained this family in some dark secret had been removed from
everyone in the room. One by one they all sat down and began
touching him.

His bed became an altar and he the sacrifice that became eternal
life. A story was written that day whose specifics I'll never know. But
I was witness to a true healing far beyond anything my ventilator or
my antibiotics could have offered. It's been twenty-five years, and
that story is still written on my soul.

Three Themes

These stories touch on three themes we should keep in mine if we
intend to honor the soul's legacy in this world. First, *what we intend
to give may have very different impacts than we realize.* An embattled
Medicare patient of mine once said, "These are the golden years. It
takes a lot of gold to get through them." The last of a life may squan-

der all the riches that lifetime was devoted to accruing. Families come to blows over the inheritance; a child's dreams are chained to a family business he feels he must carry on; the "deathbed promise" may prove a stake through a loved one's heart.

Second, *each gift is the beginning of a very, very long exchange.* Jorge Luis Borges told a tale of lives transformed by books delivered "C.O.D." to the bereaved at a series of funerals. The children and friends have their worldview transformed when they discover that the saintly uncle was ordering pornography, the nasty old drunk read religious and philosophical texts, or the recluse exchanged books with friends all over the world. The emotionally remote brother read poetry! Families were enriched, disrupted, destroyed by the spreading waves of realization.

In the end, the teller discovers that a corrupt bookseller is fraudulently sending bundles of old books to funerals he finds in the newspaper. The books have no relationship to the individuals. Yet the books take on a life that extends beyond, becomes more real, than the deceased.

Or did Borges intend to explore the notion that the lie mysteriously, intuitively captured the deeper essence of the person? Did the unknown schemer speak for the soul? We can help families and patients create stories that make that life a permanent feature on the map of their worlds; we have immense power to determine precisely what story we help them create and how each story speaks to those of us who were present.

The third point is that we honor most deeply not by transforming or fantasizing about the loved one but by *cherishing her for her true nature.* Our society loves the luminescence of beauty, wealth, or power. When we deny the darkness, that in us which is humble or wounded, we discard much of what we came here to be. I have seen patients so worried about their stock portfolios, their tax dodges, and the King Lear–like division of their bequests that their last days drowned in struggle and resentment. Family feuds tore open wounds the end of a life could have healed.

It's possible that this preoccupation with the worldly, and even the passing down of the obsessions and sicknesses that occupied a life, could be interpreted as honoring the (sadly decrepit) essence of the individual. But it's my suspicion that this is rather a continuation of a lifelong pattern of denying the soul.

Midwives to the Myth

Like two gametes that form a zygote in one cell, events become a living entity through the mixing of distinct views and interpretations, through the maturing processes of time and reflection. The entity is shaped by every blow, every shout and drug that buffet it in the womb. And finally, at a time of abrupt turmoil and pain, it is brought into the light. Every other aspect of the soul—its denial, its calling, the uniqueness of the individual, the eternal and the universal—is experienced by the living as the legacy the departing soul plants in us.

We who work with the last of life are the story's midwives. We boil the water that will clean things up. We shuffle around doing important and irrelevant busywork so everyone will know we cared. We arrange the scene so events can unfold in the most auspicious manner. We shape the story in the dim light of flickering candles that represent the warming or scarring embers of an ancient hearth.

Jan Bernard wrote in *The True Work of Dying,*

> The dying process has its own rhythms of care: repositioning a body through massage and gentle shifts, swabbing the mouth that is parched from lack of fluids, and holding and talking to the one you love as the body moves closer to death. The pregnant woman's body contracts to push the baby out of the womb. In the labor of the dying one, the contractions are the progressive shutting down of the body, literally pushing the spirit out from within it. The body loses the ability to move, it can no longer regulate its own temperature. The ability to eat or drink is gone. A person can no longer do anything without help—except leave the body.

... The skill of midwifing may mean stepping back and getting in touch with past instincts and memories. As Elisabeth Kübler-Ross teaches, it involves listening and being attuned to the dying one. Being a midwife may mean being fully oneself.

... When our eyes met, I saw the same clarity in her eyes that I saw in women giving birth. It was a look that comes only from suffering. It seemed as though she could see into my very soul. I remembered what Elisabeth Kübler-Ross had said about being completely honest with your patients, so I shared with Ellen my fears, my uncertainty about caring for her. She smiled at me and said, "Come sit with me until I fall asleep." It was then that I moved from my head to my heart and followed her guidance about what to do, rather than trying to figure it out on my own.

These descriptions capture two essential features: how we prepare to be delivered from this life and body into what follows, and how profoundly caregivers are touched, created, even reborn by the deaths we attend.

If we are assisting not just in the release of the soul but in the birth of a myth that will survive in this world, what tools do we have to become such coauthors?

I would look to the births of my two children.

Joshua Fischer Bartlow was born February 25, 1991, after forty-four hours of labor. He was so large he required cesarean section. When his head popped out, we thought he was Samoan. His eyes opened immediately, looking at each of us piercingly. When he was handed to his mother, she said, "Oh, my beautiful boy, all the girls are going to love you!"

Maya Fischer Bartlow was born June 22, 1995. Her biologic mother came up from Mexico carrying a child for whom she'd concluded she could not care. Gabriela was so brave, we all forgot to provide her any pain relief. I tried to deliver Maya, but her shoulders were very broad; another man had to guide her out. Maya came into the world in a rush of water, slick as if she'd been training to come here all her life. Within a minute, she was in her brother's lap; the wonder and joy in his eyes filled the entire world.

Years later, these stories still define how I and my children interpret their paths. Joshua embodies largeness, the long struggle, clarity and beauty. Maya's days are filled with her easy naturalness in the world, her broad, determined shoulders, the help from friends where her parents won't suffice, and her brother's cosmic love.

Had it gone differently, or had we focused on the things that fell short, we might feel differently about them, about the world, about ourselves. Perhaps even today, the ways we felt we'd fallen short limit the health and potential of our children. The myth creates the reality.

The Tools of the Storyteller's Craft

Physical

Set the material world right. Change the names on the bank accounts. Assign Durable Power. Settle the will.

Create the environment in which a "home death" can best proceed. Bring together the objects, words, and people who will make it feel right. Allow them time and quiet space in which to work their healing magic.

Be honest and clear about the medical prognosis, the burdens of therapies, and the quality of likely outcomes. We can decide whether death will be one final deception or the setting aright of all that wasn't true in this life.

Meaning

What is the significance of this life, this illness, and this death? What does it tell those who remain here about the world we live in and how to live in it? Does the story ennoble us or make us feel small and weak? Is it a story about safety or danger? Is it about failure or victory? Every life and death can be told in all these different ways. We begin by acknowledging that we are attending to the meaning of the life and death.

Purpose

Why did I come here? Why is each of us here in this room? What do we need to do? What calls out to be healed? And once known, how will we heal it? Here, now, in this room, each of this nearly random batch of struggling beings has come with a purpose that can and must be honored.

Creative Memory

This is both the result and the method of recognizing the physical, philosophical, and teleological aspects of the last of life. Positive memories can frame the illness and begin the healing of the next generations. Memories are the brick and mortar of the legacy. Searing, painful memories become misdirected into lawsuits at insensitive doctors and guilt over not protecting a loved one better than we did. There's no healing there, only more abuse.

Which part of the events we choose, which of the reactions we weigh as real, are the raw stuff from which the story will grow? Each minute of each part of the end of a life is an opportunity to shape those memories. The soul's intention may be revealed more by motive than by actual outcomes. An ethical battle born of love and compassion may heal both the soul departing and those left behind. An ethical battle born of fear and envy may cripple souls on both sides.

Emotion

"Facts inform. Stories enlighten." Many different belief systems concur: heaven sounds so great, what in God's name did we bother to come here for? Surely an all-powerful God wouldn't drop us into this mess just out of sardonic humor, would she? What did we come here to experience? Well, it's hard to find a better source of emotion than the last of a life. Our final days should be chock-full of humor, misery, confessions of fallibility, tears of regret, flashes of anger, and admissions of unimaginably brutal alienation. Our society tends to smother death beneath heavy shrouds of dishonesty and artifice. Yet it is in the final days that we find the last, best opportunity to "get real."

The unleashing of emotions is the very core of the storyteller's art.

After

We call it grief therapy, grieving groups, last rites, sitting shivah, requiem. It's the denouement, the "untying the knot" that gives a shape to all the loose ends. Under all these guises, it is how we rationalize and emotionally honor the story of a life; the sooner we do so, the better for all of us. When I was a child in Omaha, some minister had his wake before he died; he didn't want to miss all the fun and good food, and besides, he wanted to hear what they were going to say about him. By giving the legacy a seat in the room, right next to the chair where Death waits impatiently, we all get to write our stories together.

Two days before Jay died, I walked in on a painful face-off. For the first time, I met A.J., whose lifelong bitterness at his father and everything about his world was in the process of blowing sky high. Jay was lecturing him about Jesus and how much easier things were for his son than they were for him. On the other side of the mirror, A.J. was ranting about all the people who were bringing him down, controlling him, wrecking his life just like his father had. I was watching four million years of fathers and sons, each talking at the other in a foreign tongue.

I asked A.J. to think about what he'd like his dad to carry away with him—what lesson, what forgiveness, what memory. And I suggested that Jay consider what he'd want to remember as his role in the last of his time in this world. Both of them looked at me as if I had taken a wrong turn at another planet. But Jay thought for a while, then offered, "I was a hard father and did too much being angry and drinking too much. It wasn't easy for any of them. But now I feel so easy. I know they love me, no matter what I did."

A.J. sat studying his tattooed forearms, his hands clenching into fists as his dad seemed to drift between attention and an amused reverie of some more lovely place. The son looked at me with fear in his eyes. "I feel like a well and the cap is about to blow off." Angie watched both warily, tears welling up that this long lifetime of resentments filled the room even at the end. Not exactly by her choice, she'd been given three years to work through the hurts between herself and her father. But her brother had avoided it all, and it was crashing in on him.

I was writing this chapter in this book about the legacy; it made me think differently than I might have otherwise. "That cap blowing off may be the greatest gift your dad's death can give you. It's opening you up to all the hurt and loss your anger has tried to keep away. If you want to honor what your dad's trying to do now, how he's trying to make up for all the trouble he caused you and you caused him, your work will be to keep that cap off."

I found myself thinking for a minute of some of the people who had been so generous in helping me to learn about the last of life. Hospice workers, volunteers, and dying patients have taught me a word I still barely understand: grieving. They've talked of grieving groups and healing. Christina, my editor, ran bereavement groups for parents who had lost children. Grieving. Bereavement. I always thought they just meant sadness and something to do with black crape.

But in that room I became aware of Angie's hoping with her whole heart for the best for her dad and brother. I became aware of how deep and how high is the raging pressure in that well of loss we each carry. I even felt that cap in myself trying to blow.

"I don't know you, A.J., and I don't know your struggles. Your dad can't undo how he hurt you in the years past. But maybe you can use this to keep the lid off so your angers and fears can be released.

The Hospice group here does grieving groups for people who have lost loved ones. It's not all sadness; there's a lot of joy and guilt, anger, and getting lost so you can find your way back home. I've met some of them; they're good people who have been through what you're maybe ready to do.

"You can decide what to take from your dad's death. There's something in you you're furious at. Maybe his death can help you find it and let it go."

Jay cut in: "Son, I let my anger hurt too many people. I don't want you to make the same mistakes." Angie had told her brother that she thought he was enraged at himself because he had no control over their dad and hadn't been able to protect his sister and mother from him. How, he wondered, could she know?

My brief time with the family was over. Jay's legacy will weave through the rest of their lives. Angie tells me how joyful she is that she dared spend those last couple of years making her peace with her dad. It was actually the day he decided to stop dialysis that she felt the resentments slip away and began having flashbacks to the bonds of healing, honesty, and forgiveness that had formed between them. So many wounds had become unimportant, and the love between them had returned from wherever love hides and refuses to die.

From the experience, Angie came to realize what a "gift of love" is in her. It had been there in her work years before with battered women and rape-crisis intervention; it had been there for her children; but now she is aware of how it permits her to forgive and to connect. She tells her children stories that flow from her father: how she'll not spank them because she'll "lose control" as her father did. How brother and sister should cherish one another, need one another, and share. How it's okay for a son to have feelings and a daughter to demand not to be abused.

She remembers the lessons of this time of illness and death. "Life isn't about going to work and getting a paycheck. It's about what we go to work for—connection, love, and what we want to do.

"I have to take life as it comes. When bad stuff comes down, I find myself asking not 'Why me?' but 'What am I supposed to learn from this, now?'"

A.J. went home and poured his heart out to his wife. They're opening up, planning to do some kind of therapy together. He needed to see his dad break down, lose control—this time not into rage but into tears. It didn't happen, but the tears that flowed at last were A.J.'s. Angie thinks we each yearn to see in our parents what they're most afraid of revealing—their humanity. A.J.'s family is at the beginning of a dangerous journey, and it may or may not end happily. But Jay's death offered his son a place farther along the road than his father had been able to go before his illness. At the memorial service, A.J. confessed that he had not honored his father. Each day that he chooses to follow the teaching and love Jay offered him at the end, he does the greatest honor to the spirit that lives on and may be watching.

Jay went down a checklist of his life. He reviewed the beginning, middle, end. He had conversations he'd long neglected and psychic conversations with those who weren't present. When Angie challenged him about this, he smiled cagily and pointed to his mind. Somewhere in there, the sense of abuse and defenselessness was released.

A few hours before Jay's death, there was a scene neither of his children thought they'd ever see. He went from somnolent to vibrantly alert. His former wife, their mother, was visiting. She and Jay had taken to talking again after a decade of cruel silence. They went down the hall to share a smoke, and Jay said he was deeply sorry for all the hurt he'd caused. She denied that the blame was all his to bear alone. She'd done her share to drive him up the wall, just for spite. They talked for hours and shared some good nostalgic laughs.

I can feel Jay smiling somewhere that his death achieved what his life had never gotten around to. He'd come home to a family that he loved and that loved him. They'd work it out together.

The popularity of the theme song from the film *Titanic* captures how much we each need to feel that life and love don't end with death: "I believe that the heart will go on and on." The character Rose says, "And so now you know there was a man named Jack Dawson, and that he saved me in every way it is possible for a person to be saved."

This is the power each dying person has. They can bequeath to us who survive, and carry on into eternity, the knowledge that their death healed us, transformed us, opened doors that we thought were closed forever.

EIGHTEEN

The Soul as Manifestation of the "One": We All Come to Be Healed

God knows, I was not in the mood to give psychological explanations or to preach any sermons—to offer my comrades a kind of medical care of their souls. I was cold and hungry, irritable and tired, but I had to make the effort and use this unique opportunity. ... I told them of a comrade who on his arrival in camp had tried to make a pact with Heaven that his suffering and death should save the human being he loved from a painful end. For this man, suffering and death were meaningful; his was a sacrifice of the deepest significance. He did not want to die for nothing. None of us wanted that. ... Only too rarely had I the inner strength to make contact with my companions in suffering and ... I must have missed many opportunities for doing so.

—Viktor Frankl,
Man's Search for Meaning

*M*OST CAREGIVERS DISGUISE their own fears and isolation as a "need for objectivity." We find it particularly hard to touch the part of ourselves that dies with each patient. Sadly, the caregiver who hides his own fears of mortal loss, her own deepest questions, behind layers of important busyness becomes little more than an empty white coat.

Preoccupied with what we have to offer others, we have no training in recognizing the gifts each dying patient can infuse into *us* if given the chance. But when we dare that disquieting journey, suddenly our patient regains his power to touch all of us around him, and we honor his soul, all of our souls, most deeply. I've come to believe that it is in the soul as *One* that the seed of true healing resides.

The key to meeting the soul as *One* is *acceptance*, but an acceptance much broader than simply accepting someone else's disease or death. We must begin by accepting our own mortality, our own weakness and need. We must be ready to reach out for help. This patient, this family, have been taken to their most essential depths by the force of an illness or impending death. We must be ready to accept the love and wisdom they offer us in so precious a moment, or we pick a pointless death over vibrant life.

Apart

When death approaches in the hospital, a chill runs through us all. The air changes, the routines of the day become confused between cure and care, the doctors' visits become more perfunctory because we don't really have many numbers or plans to report. We nod sadly, discuss the adequacy of excretory function, and beat a hasty retreat.

In that gaping silence looms the shadow of what needs to be spoken.

My predominant experience of hospitals, with all the staff bustling around each patient, is the tremendous isolation we each feel. Nurses pull together as ward groups and do grow remarkably close to the patients and families, but they're taught not to look at their own needs and wounds. Whatever they suffer is considered just part of the territory. They're there to support, to give of themselves. Therapists run all over the place; the administrators are stashed away in the fancy suites downstairs, cut off from those they would serve.

The family has a waiting room as far from the doctors' lounge as geography will permit, and the doctors withdraw to their private offices, where they take refuge in a thousand other demands.

Our "professionalism" is built on a scientific model of objectivity. But the separation of object and subject is rapidly revealing itself to be an illusion, as shown by numerous experiments mentioned earlier. Health care providers are touched in a powerful but secret way by every person for whom we care. When one patient is dying, something is dying and being opened up in every one of us. When we put a patient through a pointless trauma, we are all traumatized. When one is healed, we are all anointed with the sweet herbs of healing.

It is worth asking, What draws caregivers to our profession? What is it in us that yearns to be cared for? What questions do we come to the fields of illness and death to have answered?

Rachel Remen wrote clearly and beautifully in *Kitchen Table Wisdom* of the wages we reap when we close ourselves off from the wealth of human experience. She described one elderly professor who sadly admitted that for all his honors and acclaim, he reached the end of his career knowing nothing more about life than he did at the beginning. Another, an oncologist, feeling he had "nothing more" to offer his patient, suggested they pray. He wasn't religious, he didn't even know how to go about it, but they got to their knees, and she healed him.

Einstein studied physics to learn how God thought. Carl Sagan, one of the great rationalists of our time, wrote of a godless universe that seems holy, unified, and intentional. Yet we at the bedside turn from the waves of feeling that wash over us all every day. That person in the bed, alone, going through an individual death, is being distilled into spirit and universal experience. She is going where we all will go. As parts of her self are stripped away, deeper realities are revealed to each of us.

Yet we caregivers around her deny that it has anything to do with us.

One Is Dying for All

She has lost her independence, her place in the world. She reveals to us how dependent, needy, scared we ourselves feel.

Control of her life and fate have fallen into our hands. She can show us what it is to live without the illusion of control.

She seems impotent. We can discover what our essential power is—to touch others without coverings, to face deep truths, to reveal ourselves. When nothing we thought mattered remains, we can reach for what truly does matter.

She is terrified, adrift, out of control. We can see that part of ourselves that feels this way and through that fearsome rent in our façade know what we are most afraid of losing. What is this essence that the more tightly held, the more rapidly slips from our grasp?

She is dying away before our eyes. What do we feel dying within ourselves? What needs to die—our possessiveness, our anger, our doubts? Our isolation? She is becoming a vibration barely recognizable. What resonance is our soul prepared to receive?

She looks so alone there in the bed. Around her are children and other family members and all of us. But it's as if she's in a bubble of a death she alone is experiencing. We can sense just how alone we each feel. The near-death reports of long-lost friends and family welcoming us at the other end of the tunnel touch each of us deeply: they suggest that the end of isolation is a heavenly reward we've long sought. This coming together is part of what is missing in this life of ours, so busily crowded with other solitary souls.

Are we really so distinct, so alone? Perhaps we're really emissaries sent here to bring news back to the universal. Are we all fingers reaching out from one vast body? Feeling the deep upheaval this death causes within us, we can recognize that we're each an integral part of every other being.

What this patient is experiencing is happening in each of us. It is happening in the old man staggering down the street outside with his bottle in a paper bag. It is in the plant wilting on the windowsill and the cars stirring up dust in the street outside, and in the scarred hills out beyond the city's edge.

Barriers to the Universal

What makes us flee these deep oceans of experience? For one thing, we have spent our whole lives seeing ourselves as distinct, as autonomous units. If we are only physical beings, which is all science can prove, then death is nothing but our final, terrifying dissolution. It's too uncomfortable to face.

Yet we caregivers have placed ourselves in death's presence for some reason. The question is whether we will be here openly and wisely, or falsely and closed to our own purpose. The germ theory of disease encourages us to wash our hands between cases so we don't spread the dis-ease around. Unfortunately, we treat spirit the same way: if we absorb too much in this room, it will burden us in the next. If we open to our own yearnings and panic, our existential pain, we'll be unable to "be there" for the next patient. I've found over the past few years that the exact opposite is true. When we open to one patient, we're more resonant to all, more astute, more insightful. The wound that is opened in us by one patient's struggles and resurrection opens our spirits to all of those around and within us.

We are frightened by the power of the soul's demand that we face our own darkness. To know that we will die, that all we hold dear will fall from us, that our possessions and status are only of the moment, brings into question the value of everything we do. The soul is calling, "You've come here to learn, to experience intimacy, to let go of the trappings that give you a false security. You came to be with this person who is dying, not for your hourly wage or another entry on your curriculum vitae or so you could buy another car. You came here because through the way you are with him, and he with you, you will manifest parts of yourself that your ego has denied you."

As a life wanes, every mood it feels washes over us. And like it or not, we carry those feelings to the next room, and the next day, and home to our families. There are patients whose depression is so deep or their need so profound that I dread walking into their presence. Yet if I can feel through them the depth of my own emptiness and yearning, I can begin to heal these wounds within me. The patient has tendered me a gift. I choose every day, every instant, whether to receive it.

The Soul We Bury Before the Death

In our denial of this offering, these parts of our patients most inimical or mysterious to us, we bury the patient long before his death arrives to take him. I remember a man named John, a brilliant architect who had the bad habit of getting stoned and drawing water from the toilet for the heroin he injected into his veins. How's that for a soul statement of how he felt about himself? Anyway, as usual, his seizure dragged me out of my call room at three A.M., which in no way inclined me to appreciate him. He was just another druggie, wildly demanding, seizing and despairing and ringing the call bell every two minutes. He had a devoted companion who assailed me with demands for information, answers I didn't have, reassurances I wasn't about to fabricate. Always they wanted more and more and more attention. More. They were demanding what I least felt like giving.

We eventually drained the abscess from his brain and got him cleaned up. When the seizures stopped he became compliant in a screwy, offhanded sort of way. Rather against my own wishes, I actually started liking him. I started thinking maybe I could save him from his life of drugs. His family was brilliant but with an undercurrent of abuse and alcoholism, and it hurt to think how the threads of family and experience invisibly wove through our daily misdeeds. His work was as well respected and unique as mine, his hopes perhaps not much different from my own. Yet here he was trapped in the bed with a huge zipper carved into the side of his scalp, while I stood to the side, my beeper tearing me away from any real contact.

As he improved, I moved on to other patients. Then one day I noticed a dozen sketches taped to his wall. They were in heavy pencil; there was about them the same unrepentant, raw urgency I'd seen in scrimshaw remnants from concentration camps where people had risked their lives to carve something that would document their experience and prove they had lived. John's drawings were of him in the bed, of us coming in and out like avenging angels, his companion stooping over him, John as an archangel, a brilliant light with concerned shadows around it (this was years before the first "near-death" reports). I was stunned at the beauty and foreboding power of his work. I encouraged him to do more and suggested we could do a book about the "concentration camp" aspects of a serious illness. From the moment I suggested that, he never drew another picture as far as I was aware. He "recovered," left the hospital, and was dead a year later of complications from recurrent drug use.

For years I've kicked myself for not getting those pictures out of him before he died. But as I write this all these years later, John is still alive in me. I realize words such as *attention, concentration, alive, dark* fill the commentary. Trying to get his pictures for a book was just another effort to get something physical to hold on to, to prove I was still alive and in control. But his true gift was to draw my attention, to force my concentration on himself. He succeeded, and decades later he reminds me how much each patient has to teach me, if only I'll pay attention. The pictures were only one of the gimmicks, a technique patients' souls have available to touch our souls as our technology consumes their bodies.

Another patient may grab us through his complaints and crazy acting out. Or I may discover something ancient in the wrinkles of a hand and the cool, knobby bones beneath. An old lady's eyes sink under their lids like slippery frogs beneath a pair of soft leaves. Their movement is so slight, it's not clear there's any movement left. The particular way she picks at her blankets reminds me of picking away the layers of confusion to find the treasures beneath.

The man over there grumbles and rumbles as he moves from his bed to the commode, implacable and huge as some crude lava flow shifting the core of the earth.

They grab us, make us bear witness that a real person is here, someone like ourselves who's hurting and isolated, in love with a particular set of fantasies, scared, exuberant, determined, yielding, and adrift all at the same time. It's then that they can teach us whatever we've come to learn.

When we open our patients to questions of the soul, we prepare to listen to our own. When we ask them what it means to them to die, and what they expect will follow death, our own soul is asking. We who practice in this world close to death must be reminded by those closer to death what life is here to do. Dying patients, given the chance to touch us, can awaken our deadness by the vitality and clarity that fills them.

～

Jay wound down like a record playing its last tune, sometimes stuck in a groove. He again told Angie, "He's my best friend." They're words I've hungered for my whole life. Yet the things we most want are those we most doubt we will ever deserve.

He saw in me a capacity for caring that often gets lost in my preoccupations and irritations. He saw beyond failings and absences to a person who heard him openly. As his heart opened, he opened mine. In a perpetual commerce, what other patients had given me helped carry Jay through his last part of this earthly journey.

We had a remarkable final few days. The local paper was doing a series on the end of life. I'd worked with the health reporter, Thom Gabrukeiwicz, on some of the themes, and now they wanted to take pictures. At the last minute, I realized the blatantly obvious: that this story should be about patients, not doctors. Jay's and my picture made it to the front page along with his story. The Sunday lead article would come out two days after his transfer to a nursing home for terminal care.

Saturday evening he called, asking to restart dialysis so he could survive long enough to see the series; he'd come to take immense pride in showing how the decision to end life support could be made with courage and peacefulness. He wanted to "glorify the Lord's name." He felt people "want to have hope for a continuing existence," and that his story might help confirm that.

Instead of my arranging dialysis, Angie called the paper, and late Saturday night Thom spirited the galley proofs across town so the star of his article could study the series. Both were pleased, and I'm told he and Angie spent some long hours together that night in and out of tears.

Weeks later, people were coming up to me on the street and saying, "Aren't you that bald guy on the front of the paper? I read that article; it was a great piece." Some of them were elderly, some ill, some teenagers! Jay's legacy lives on with them, and in Thom, in generations of children and family, and in me. I believe his eternal spirit was touched by those who cared about him. He knew his choices were honored and the meaning of his life was rewritten by how he chose to pass his final hours.

He will live in me the rest of my time, reminding me. He reminds me that I too will have the chance to choose my death and to create the last of my life. I too am filled with love and yearning, if only I will take the cap off the well. I have been taken as the best of friends and been offered the best of friendship many times in this amazing swirl of caring that is life together on the planet. Jay's path can guide me and, through me, all for whom I care.

Angie gave me at the end one more gift of "the soul as *One*." When she spoke of what my friendship had meant to Jay, I asked if she and her father had known how deeply I had been touched by their feelings about me. She said, "No," as if it were a ridiculous question. Certainly we caregivers wound ourselves to the core by denying our own need for a healing touch. But beyond that, when we fashion ourselves as invulnerable heroes, givers who will not receive, we deny our patients the joy of knowing that they too are our healers. Part of every death is regret; it is how we learn, how we become through loss more than we were before. My regret with Jay is that I kept from him all he had inspired in me. This book is in large part a testimonial, an act of gratitude, to all those who live within me still and a wish that I could have had the courage to let them know how profoundly they had touched me.

Mirrored in the grace of each death, I am discovering the fullness of my life. Opening my heart to the beauty and internal wisdom of the lives others have lived, I begin to perceive the purpose that will shape my life and my death.

Through all time, these many souls and mine will be *One*.

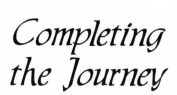

PART FIVE

Completing the Journey

*D*o you know why the bamboo is here? It is
waiting for the wind's touch. It is full of
emotion. Listen: you can hear it.

—from the motion picture, *Red Corner*

NINETEEN

As I Lay Dying: Completing Life Through Illness and Death

Preparation

So now I am dying. Perhaps this time it will be for good.

Death, it turns out, isn't some sudden disaster that rips a life apart. Quite the opposite. Most of a century ago, I was born full of wisdom and purpose, full of the spirit of what had been before this life. Yet even before birth, bits of me had begun dying. I had to give up a yolk sac to make a stomach. Gills and a tail fell away so I could one day breathe and walk.

The first thing I lost was my memory of that other place of clear light. Descending into my body, I felt myself surging down my spine, from spirit to vision, through the will that secretly and stubbornly would occupy the years ahead. I entered the world screaming my absolute determination to *be!* This wondrous heart of mine was pulsing against my mother's passage—this heart I had come here to experience. As I struggled to be born, I felt churning in my belly the infant urge to control everything around me. At some place lower down in me was the knowledge that I was here to create and conceive, to be an instrument of learning. A thread of energy was about to connect me to this earth and this conscious "reality" for the intermezzo of one brief human existence.

Many times in the life that followed, I would lose contact with my soul's purpose. The fear would arise that I'd never have power or get what I imagined I needed. I would tremble when I feared that I would fall short of my dreams. During many dark nights, this journey seemed so hopeless that my tenuous connection to my earthly existence nearly broke. One less breath, one more moment of pain or disappointment, and I would have drifted away. But none of those deaths of the spirit became a physical death. None until this one.

A Stone in the River

Nearly a decade ago, a pain hit just below my shoulder blade. My wife looked at me with an expression of concern I hadn't seen before: Was it my heart? Was it cancer? Though we didn't discuss the new worry that had just entered our lives, we finally found time to prepare our Advance Directives. As it turns out, I've been able to express my wishes to the end—but looking at such questions back then made us consider what we had left to complete in whatever life remained. For the first time I was forced to evaluate what mattered most. I had battled for years on end to create a hundred illusions of myself—status, authority, power, always being right—that I wanted others to see and acknowledge. As each of these illusions slipped away, I would discover how untrue, how limiting each presumption had been. My anger at my children and friends, I realized, had been nothing more than love wasted and hours I would never retrieve.

These dear souls I presumed were so close to me didn't know what to do when I began laying aside my harshness and reaching out to them, one by one. Admittedly, I did so awkwardly. But gradually they accepted that I was undergoing some kind of transformation. With grace and incredible courage, they opened themselves to me whenever I became able to let them into my heart. It was strange: I was the one the x-rays and lab specimens said was dying, but we all began to come to life. Politics, religion, lifestyles, all the things to which we attached such importance and that kept us apart, revealed themselves as utter trivia. Before, when I started to feel too close to another person, I would become uneasy and muster my forces for a confrontation, or just retreat into silence. When I glared at a threatening "loved one," it was if I saw them hidden behind an obscuring mirror. Now it was different. The part of me that knew my time was short reached out and broke the glass; we each suddenly discovered on the other side unknown, yearning beings crafted of our own flesh.

Looking for another adversary, I turned my rage on this damned condition that was killing me. I was as determined to destroy my disease as it was to eat out my insides. I considered the illness another of the many ways my life had cheated me. I've struggled with it, hated it, and destroyed myself trying to beat it. But at the end of these years of battle, we've made a peace of sorts, and the illness has reciprocated by nudging my roots ever deeper into the earth like some great oak reaching toward the limits of its span. Released from fear and resentment, how far can I reach? How long can my meaning survive?

Faced with this illness, I was forced to decide what I wanted to leave my children and my wife. I even began thinking about religion. What would be left of me after I departed this life? Was there eternity? The illness gave me time to examine all these questions. I began remembering again. I was given the first glimmerings that what I'd come here to achieve didn't involve money or power or control. The best of my legacy would be not things but ideas and memories. And beyond the words, I might leave healing embraces offered just in the nick of time.

It's Time

Today may be the day I'll die. Though they'll not say it, it's clear that nothing my physicians and nurses can do will restore me to a quality of life I would find worthwhile. Over these few years, I've thought of many of these dedicated but somehow locked-down caregivers as everything from saviors and saints to assailants and dupes. This time when they were talking at me, their eyes revealed that they were far more lost and confused than I, the one who was supposed to be help-lessly dying. They had come to their scientific profession full of childlike trust, like believers on pilgrimage to Lourdes in pursuit of the healing waters. Today's would-be healers do not understand that they come to hospital bedsides seeking their own cure. My hospital bed has become a little shrine where the waters flow in and out of polystyrene tubes but offer those through whom they pass precious little benefit. Too often these waters stave off death but do nothing to nourish the soul. Too often those who come to heal have, through their very training and science, been robbed of the words required to reach out in supplication and find what they are really searching for in this life. Now at the hour of my death they gather at my bed-side to support me, which inspires a sort of bemused awe. But I've begun to see so much more.

I see their fear, their helplessness and nakedness before the dark, unnamed stranger who sits in the corner chair, escorting me through the last of this life. They don't see him. Or perhaps he's too immense and obvious for them to acknowledge. I realize that all these would-be healers are seeking, hoping for something when they come to my bedside, but they don't know what it is or how to ask it of me.

Still, their uneasiness makes me feel less alone. Now I can sense my life growing narrower, confined to this bed, as time expands. The present reaches out to embrace an entire life that was never lived in the present. It welcomes home the time before this existence and the eternity that will follow. I have begun what I've read is called the "true work of dying." I hope that all the petty grievings for a long life's innumerable losses will have prepared me for this final griev-ing as I turn one large loss into what needs to be one true meaning.

Home: The Connection to Earth

How I wish I could be in my own bed. The folks who care for me are working on that. Until then, this naked room with all its clicking monitors and staff rushing in and out will have to be as much of a home as we can make it. On TV I've seen primitive people who paint themselves, hop around in a frenzy, wail, and tear out their hair to express their grief. Here they get themselves up in ridiculous vestments of masks and sterile gowns, scurry in and out, and work until they drop. Little green iridescent lines bleep out the drumbeats. In the midst of such meaningless, unrelenting rites, how shall I make this a home?

I need my family and friends really close to me now. When they're here, they shuffle about, sit around pained and restless, trying to figure out what not to say. Well, I say this: let's welcome Death and put him in a chair of his own; grant him his name, then get on with the remains of the day. Do we have so much time left to waste in charades? Let's talk as we used to. Reminisce, tell the stories that always made us laugh! What's so wrong with a bit of laughter? I'd like to have—oh, let's see—some of my pictures over there, and somebody to stroke the guitar I always had in my office but forgot how to play, and some books. Books always took me back into myself. My wife and I slept under a comforter that always made me feel as if I were nestled in her breasts. I'd like that, and my own pillow. If I were an animal person, I'd ask you to put our dogs in my lap when I die. Alas, I wasn't. Those rowdy beasts competed too much for the affection I thought I needed. So I'll have to settle for a book or two. My mind imagines the smell of black fur and warm, earthy breath nuzzling devotion into my ear. Perhaps in the next life I'll be brave enough to let the animals come in.

How many afternoons meandered toward the sunset with our music playing in the background? The music has been missing. And the most precious music of all: when I was admitted to the hospital, those in charge wouldn't let our grandchildren play around my feet. More died in me that day than is about to die. Please get the music and the music of their voices back into my room.

Though I can't swallow anymore, I would love one last time to have the taste of that special stew of yours on my tongue. And I yearn to be touched. It seems as if everyone's become afraid to touch me, except to turn me and change the sheets and the dressings and pat powder in all those places I never would have let a stranger mess with before. How I loved the caresses, holding hands, the macho nonsense of slaps on the shoulder, the sense of curling around my wife's spine through the long night. I've lost them all: I'd like them back now. I'm not radioactive. I'm not some fragile porcelain. I will soon blow away like ash in the wind, but I'm not gone yet. My death is not contagious: it's life and love that are catching.

When time grows short, it takes on a remarkable meaning. During my life, I was a slave to time; I struggled for time; I was always battling someone for control of my time. My wife drove me crazy by having people drop in any time of the day or night. She loved the chaos and festivity of an open door, and we fought about it. I didn't realize until now that she was trying to open the door to a closed-off part of myself, to shout at me, "The whole world's out here! Come and join the party!" Home is a place where people can drop by anytime, stay as long as they wish, and go at their leisure. It's a place where we can relish one another's presence, savoring one another's company like watching beautiful autumn leaves drifting past a window. Now the little time that remains to me is once again out of my control. Please get these jailers to put away their petty schedules and rounds and "visiting time is over." If I don't get to have my own way now, when will I?

What a curious assortment of characters flutters about my room! Here are the people who have filled my life—my family, my friends. But they're all mixed in with strange, uniformed beings who have come to shepherd me out of life. The doctors, the nurses, and the therapists keep running off to the ward clerk, who seems to keep this Rube Goldberg contraption running. My heart warms to that one housekeeper who's taken a particular interest in me. She says I remind her of her father. Not likely, but I'll take what I can get. She's the one who makes me feel the best about the whole circus. She sweeps around the bed and dumps the trash, but it feels as if she's cleaning all the cobwebs out of my soul.

There's a time when you know you're either on your way out of the hospital or out of the world. I've seen it down the hall a dozen times. It's when the social worker starts inquiring about dozens of burdensome arrangements and the chaplain becomes unusually en-couraging and profound. When he starts talking about the meaning of it all, you know your goose is cooked. These ancillary presences tell me what the doctors won't. It's as if they've come to hang up lovely lace curtains and fluff the spiritual pillows. But something of their humanity leaks through the cracks in the rituals. Something like empathy between them and me accidentally opens the window to a heady spring breeze. Their silence seems to say, "We'd all best notice it while we can."

Hurry, help me make this a home, here, now, since it's looking like this will be my last home.

Generative: The Legacy

So let me look around the room. What do I have to offer as I pre-pare to become invisible? I want to reach deep inside every one of you. Suddenly I have so much to give—a lifetime of experiences, my heart swelling with love, this newborn remembering of what it feels like to encounter the other side. I want every one of you to feel that I embraced you. Since the love so often got lost in our stuff about who was going to run whose lives, I need to tell each of you how much of your love I will carry with me.

I want you to remember me as strong and peaceful at the end but also honest about all the ways I felt my life fell short of its potential. My greatest strength would be if I could finally admit my vulnera-bility.

I'm amazed at the years I wasted in scrambling around and ob-sessing when a quiet second now could fill a library with revelations.

I want you to know I learned that lesson, and I offer that wisdom to you. There were many things I came to understand. I wish I could pass them on to you. What I value; what I wish I had been able to do; what my meaning was: "Did you get my meaning?" Well, you'd better get it now. Tomorrow will be too late.

What did I do with my life? For one thing, I always sought to excuse my pain and failures by blaming them on others. It's a family tradition: we pass such things down as surely as we do our eye color or the pigment of our skin. Someone had to be the culprit, and usually I insisted that it was one of those closest to me. And since you loved me, at least for a time, and were still open, you accepted the wounds I passed on down my family tree like bitter sap. I have much grieving to do about that, much regret to carry with me to whatever follows. For many lifetimes, you and your children will carry the marks of my fears. In this little time left, I wish I could put it right.

Years from now, I would want you to tell stories about me. Such stories are where my immortal legacy lies. It's not that I want to bind you. Rather, it's because I'd like those stories to remind you of the best of me that lives on in you and the most troublesome parts of me that you have the opportunity to reverse in yourselves.

Your eyes show so much pain and confusion. I'd like you to remember this last time as one filled with cherishing and some laughter. Let's shed some immortal amber tears over the sweetness that infused even the hardest times. Search for clarity. Demand resolution. Forgive me if you can. You need to do it. I guess my soul doesn't need to forgive; it will do whatever it needs to achieve its goals, no matter who gets hurt. But for the sake of my legacy to myself, I do forgive you all.

I'd like you to remember my last days as a source of healing. When my wife holds my hand, I want to feel again the whole world flowing between us. It's time for what flowed between me and the earth to begin passing between me and all of you. When we die, they plant us in the soil. Let my soul be planted instead in you who live on and in your time will follow me. Find in my errors cautionary tales of a man who lived too much in fear. Discover in how I'm finishing up the love I truly felt for you but couldn't express. Know you deserved it very well.

We all remember the year I brought everything down around me, every bit of my life falling in at once. God, how I despaired and cursed. I felt so worthless, abandoned by everyone, including myself. What pulled me back? Try to envision this tiny flame of curiosity deep within me. Or perhaps it was some secret belief or knowing that I had done all the harm this world would permit. Having nowhere else to turn, I knelt before the very people who are around me now. To my amazement, you lifted me up. By each of you was I lifted. You had something in you that spoke to such a part of myself. The meaning of my story would be ... No, perhaps the greatest gift I can give you is to encourage you to discover your own meaning so you can live what you needed to learn from me.

I want you to know you don't need to run from this moment. Now that the fight's over, I'm much more at ease. My gaze turns inward. For me now, your nearness fills the entire universe.

Power: Control Versus Energy

You all probably know how much of my life was a struggle for control, for domination. All of the surgeries, the powerful medications that disabled me, the radiation, even the thoughts of squirreling away enough drugs to kill myself, were just more of how I'd lived my life, trying to beat the tar out of some competitor. This time the competition was inside me, and thank God it won.

Coming to the hospital this last time banished every illusion I'd fought to preserve. I lost my clothes, my home, and any say about when or where I'd eat, even if I were able to eat. How dare they treat me this way? They even took charge of my bowels! How low can you go? But now that I have no power in the world, I begin to find incredible power in myself. When I pulled out my feeding tubes and swung them around like some kind of avenging angel, I convinced myself for an instant that I had power over my doctors with all their furiously scribbled orders and my nurses with their cajolery and threats. But in the end my heart goes out to them: they want control over us patients and our illnesses, and neither is willing to comply. It would be much better if they could let it go, as I've been forced to do, and just absorb these rich moments.

So what's become of my hallowed power? My first response to this illness was to become a teenager, rebellious and difficult, determined to do the opposite of whatever I was told. Then I was, oh, maybe six and running around doing things that made no sense and forgetting my medications, acting as if I were immortal. I nearly broke my hip falling off a ladder, painting walls that would outlive me. An IV was ticking in my shoulder and I was half stoned, but I was some kid still building his nest. Next thing I knew I was two and saying "no" to everything anybody told me to do.

Now I'm back to being a baby wailing my infinity of demands even though I can't hold a bottle to my own lips. Yet everybody is in my power, catering to my every need and trying their God-given best to dredge up some affection for this obstreperous old coot. What a trip. Even the sheets remind me of soft flannel blankets very, very long ago. And they have to change my diapers! What straits I've come to! As a doctor, I used to spout orders and throw a fit if everyone didn't hop to my demands. Now I spend hours considering whether to take a dump in the bed, just so they'll have to do something about it. Perhaps the two activities aren't all that different. How much was really about getting the job done, and how much just dumping on the nurses to feel as if I were in control?

The greatest power may be to realize what an impact I can have on every one of these people sharing my death. I recognize the power of every look, every word, to hurt or to heal. Out of the corner of my eye, I see the glimmer of a new way that is being revealed only to me. I have the power to decide when, and how, to turn toward a healing path to death. I have the power to share this knowledge with those I love and those who care for me or to keep it a secret unto myself.

This time I will use my newborn's power of all these people's con-cern for me to help each of them see what is best, what is finest in them and what is crying out to be soothed or attended to. Without lifting a finger, I have that power growing stronger in me each pass-ing second.

This time I will create, rather than be trapped by, the final scene. I will make it just right in all of our memories. When I place the comforter, have you sit here and you over there, I'm building my own afterlife as surely as Tutankhamen ever did. I will put my house in order. I will choose the room of our home from which I will de-part, or if that is not possible, re-create that room here. I will decide how much pain medication it will take for me to be peaceful. If my goal is to be alert, pain meds that dull my awareness may cause a worse pain of their own. I will decide. This time, I will not regret. Recognizing what my soul has left to complete, I will ensure that it has the space and permission to do so.

Heart of Love

We have moved beyond the silent resentments that plugged up our lives like so much rotten plumbing. Something new, barely familiar, is opening. An old cagey glance wrinkles your brow; a hesitant hand reaches out after decades of resting in your lap. Now that they real-ize Grandpa's not too busy to hold them, the grandkids sidle close. My chest feels so full sometimes that I can barely breathe. My heart beats heavy and full, but it's not from too many fluids, and it doesn't require diuretics or oxygen. It's the rich air of deep connection I've hungered for my whole life.

I've come to an ideal time to exchange a love that cherishes and laughs and is fragile yet eternal. While my body is still here, we should savor how physical that love was and how exuberantly it could dance when given the opportunity. Loving my children was a funny thing: I loved them their whole lives as they were at only one point in time—that best time, maybe when they were two or six or ten. I failed to love them as who they'd become. Or perhaps there were years when the love continued unseen like some underground river. I begin to see now that in the years when they were so uneasy with me, always angry or tense, even then there was love beneath that bitter emptiness, a love hurt and disappointed, wailing at the loss of connection. Since this is all the time I have left, what better time to recall that deep-flowing love? In words, or perhaps only in a look or a brush of fingertips, we can tell one another that the love was always there. The river will surface again to bring life to the desert. Our angers were love's champions, admittedly clumsy and foolish, but anger was not love's enemy. I never suspected how much stronger was the love than the fear that sought to protect it. The distances that grew between us are veils that need to be lifted, carefully, quickly, and with a burgeoning joy.

I think what I most appreciate in these last moments is my grandkids at the bedside. They're so much more open, so undefended. Their feelings are "out of control" in a way we all need to be. They can show their tears, and in the next instant flush with delight. They can ask without hesitation, "Grandpa, how come you smell so bad?" or, "Grandpa, are you dying?" Suddenly I smell the flowers beside the window and truly experience these children's young, vibrant lives. Then we all get to acknowledge whatever they pointed out. They're fascinated with these machines and these tubes that have gotten stuck into me. At least they're honest about their fascination. Their parents, my friends, have to sit here and pretend none of it exists. Too bad. I never thought I'd look like this at the end, but I do. So what? When my grandkids laugh or cry, they do it for everybody in the room. They and this final edition of myself have permission to show our true selves.

I love these people just now more than I ever knew I could love anything. I hope they can feel that. I hope they can let go of the old wounds, griefs, and guilts and feel what precious, vulnerable people I know have offered their lives to me. I look at them, and they almost glow. I want them to stop arguing about whether I should have more surgery, or a different medicine, or when to "give up." We give up when we're afraid to face death. That is precisely when we are afraid to face life. When we honor this work of dying that we're doing now, this joy we're experiencing now, then for the first time we don't give up.

Will: What We Came Here to Do

My throat isn't much good anymore. A tube eats for me, but I just pulled that out for good. There's a hole in my throat that breathes for me, but I've finally been heard (in a manner of speaking), so they'll not hook it to the ventilator anymore. I can barely turn my head. I have to plug the hole with this bony thumb of mine to squeeze out a few words, and even those don't seem to make all that much sense, even if you could hear them.

Yet I've never seen so clearly what I need to do and what purpose my soul had in this world. Today is my soul's destination, my destiny.

Why did I marry and have children with a woman so unlike me? Because my soul was determined to learn about connection amid chaos, about loving even when I felt unloved, about letting go of my disgusting piles of rage that drove off those I feared would abandon me. Why were acceptance and peace always just out of reach? Because I needed to learn that they were always within me, if only I would open to them. Why did I need to be special? Because I needed to realize how special is each being, each moment on this planet.

Why did my worst fears of duplicity and betrayal by others so often prove true? Because I needed to learn to trust. Why was I so often alone? Because I needed to learn that only by opening to connection with others would my life ever be genuine. The very existence of my children, their vulnerable hearts, their young lives, their open spirits kept me from fleeing to leave behind just another defeat. After so many years of evasions, they brought me into life. They were, are, and forever will be for me the meaning of love.

Just at the end do I feel the depth of the love and caring and taste the first cool waves of joy washing over us. Perhaps if I'd let them in years ago, I wouldn't even need to be sick and dying now. Or perhaps, my purpose fulfilled, I would have died back then.

Vision: Beyond Illusion

My whole world becomes this room, this home, this womb. I look at each of the people who have filled my life, or would have filled my life if I'd let them, and suddenly I see. My daughter's ridiculous choice of a man, her crazy hairdos and wild ways, were brilliant. She was searching in the world of outer pain and joy as fervently as I did in the caverns of my mind. Her courage is an act of unrelenting will. She came knowing the world was here to give her pleasure. Her flamboyant, emotional journey through some of the world's darkest places has been how she expressed her determination to find love everywhere.

My son, pondering and immobilized beside me, sits in his own personal cloud of darkness. Thinking my soul was not strong enough to heal my wounds, I passed all my worries on to him. I wish I could offer him the strength death has offered me. I would tell him, "Let these worries go. They aren't real. They have no life for you anymore. Let them go." There is a majestic light within this man. How I love him, for what he is and for the load I left him to carry.

The first suspicion that I was ill struck me a blow; I feared that now I could never become the man I had always intended to be. Surprisingly, since then my wife and I have joined in a way I couldn't have imagined. Our souls seem to sit close now, beyond words, beyond struggles, as if we were holding hands and watching the sun set on those mountains behind our house. She leans over me to kiss my body lying in this hospital bed; I catch the smells she always had about her—powder and pine and animal fur. She's so deep in the earth, I can't imagine her leaving this life in the same direction as

I. But all of that is beyond repair. I have nowhere to be but in this brief, eternal moment.

Friends sit nearby, joking and evading, debating and philosophizing. My brothers and sister reminisce about the good times when we played together. Can they hear my plea that they forgive the jealous wounds we carved into one another? Can they sense in my grip, in the way I breathe, what wondrous companions I finally realize they have been? I remember funerals with their gloomy pomp of pallbearers. My siblings, who have borne me through this long existence, must still be confused by what a stone I was in the flow of their lives. They were always there, though miles away. I was a distant, difficult man. I was a story of the wild brother far off whose return home turned everything upside down. Even now death seems only a slight way to go. That they never considered me dead, even when I did, astonishes me today as much as it did then. I hope I can give some of that gift of life back to them.

Our parents, the ancestors, all wait for me. Their eyes are so clear, as glowing as mine are soon to become. Theirs dance and laugh, run free with tears like the fresh eyes of our grandchildren. Settled as mountains, the ancient souls will become young bodies fidgeting in all this spirit work, and I know that the heart will forever go on.

Spirit: The Eternal

I'm experiencing for the second time that passage of light that connects this world to the other. In the end, each journey must be made alone. Wanting to hold on, wanting to be there, those who love us try to accompany us on the path. We must turn to them, let them know how deeply they are cherished, and encourage them to go their own way. If they persist, our vital signs stabilize, our breathing becomes easy. A few tears drift from our eyes, and the tunnel closes. But the next night or another night, when we are alone, we manage to slip away.

The top of my head is opening like a fountain. All I experienced in this life, all I brought here from before, is beginning to pour forth. I am the tunnel. I am the explorer returning with my bundle of artifacts collected in the visible world. When I was born, there was great struggle, a maelstrom of pain, and at last a releasing. Then suddenly, with a squall and a flush of vital fluids, I popped into the white sterility of a hospital. A lifetime later, I've gone through the contractions and pauses, the horrors and momentary reprieves of preparing to die. After a lifetime spent doctoring in hospitals, I will end in one. But now the walls are shimmering, transparent, and the long decades of demands and documents crumple to a mere apostrophe. Again as in birth there are loved ones around me, and again others wait for my return.

Though my eyes have lost the power to open to this illusion around me, I can perceive every one of my family and friends more clearly than I ever saw them as physical beings. Leaving this world, I feel myself coming home to those with whom I've lived, but at the same time joining those on the other side. Out at the desk, my nurses busy themselves with meaningless papers and the doctors rush back to their offices so they won't have to think of something to say, something to do when nothing they do will matter. How wrong they are. They are like farmers desperately plowing and plowing again this side of the river Styx, the river we cross into death. They think if they keep their eyes averted, the river will never come to them.

That one housekeeper comes in, leaves her pushcart for a minute or two, and stands in a corner in the shadows. It's the same corner where Death sits patiently in his own chair. She feels like a guardian angel to me now; I finally see that she is. I gesture her to my side. Barely raising two fingers, I ask her to give me her hand, so my last memory of the earth will be a human touch.

TWENTY

The Healer's Path

And the Sea will grant each man new hope, as sleep brings dreams of home.

—Tom Clancy,
The Hunt for Red October

Those of us who choose to stand close as another moves toward death will discover the deepest treasures in what we most fear, which is what we most need to love. The story goes on; it will be for another book, another time, to explore how we can reveal the healing potential of our own and our patients' souls.

I have come to believe that the true gift we offer and can receive as caregivers is to reveal the wound that inspires the healer within each of us. To do this, we must first admit how haunted we are by the memory of those we have accompanied on this passage of death, and sometimes just a bit beyond.

We must face that we are haunted by what we did or did not dare to say or feel, or do, at the end. Our fears and regrets go back to childhood, perhaps beyond that to many childhoods past. They send each of us back to the certain knowledge that I walk an uncertain but vibrant path that leads inexorably to death. I will always be surrounded by strangers empowered to determine just how I will write my last words on the stones of time.

For each of us, that haunted aching will be resolved when we realize that we will be healed not by defeating death but by honoring life so deeply that each moment draws us closer to its mysteries.

With skill and guile, with clarity and a coyote's wisdom, our souls called us here to walk toward the passage together. We must learn to cherish what the spirit calls us to do.

A river does flow between us. It's not some seething torrent that separates the living on one bank from those who are dying on the other. Rather, it's a vast and deep river that flows through all of us— all of life—the life of stones, plants, and planets. We are each born to struggle and grab a tiny toehold, to pour our substance into those dearest to us, and thereby to infuse each day with new life. It is natural and right that the river will in its time sweep us away.

I have the chance to create well the stories of my death. Others' stories of death beckon me, rich with their own lessons. A peacefulness lies ahead, as the sea waits to refresh each soul. When I let go of the fear, the love will surround me. And in that moment, I will know joy.

Bibliography

Allende, Isabel. *Paula*. New York: HarperCollins Publishers, 1994.

Bernard, Jan, and Miriam Schneider. *The True Work of Dying: A Practical and Compassionate Guide to Easing the Dying Process*. New York: Avon Books, 1996.

Bolen, Jean Shinoda. *Close to the Bone: Life-Threatening Illness and the Search for Meaning*. New York: Scribner, 1996.

Borges, Jorge Luis. *The Aleph and Other Stories, 1933–1969*. New York: E.P. Dutton, 1970.

Byock, Ira. *Dying Well: The Prospect for Growth at the End of Life*. New York: Riverhead Books, 1997.

Callahan, Daniel. *The Troubled Dream of Life: In Search of a Peaceful Death*. New York: Simon and Schuster, 1993.

Callahan, Maggie, and Patricia Kelley. *Final Gifts: Understanding the Special Awareness, Needs, and Communications of the Dying*. New York: Bantam Books, 1992.

Castaneda, Carlos. *Tales of Power*. New York: Simon and Schuster, 1974.

Chatwin, Bruce. *The Songlines*. New York: Penguin Books, 1987.

Chinen, Allan B. *In the Ever After: Fairy Tales and the Second Half of Life*. Wilmette, IL: Chiron Publications, 1989.

Chödrön, Pema. *When Things Fall Apart: Heart Advice for Difficult Times*. Shambhala, 1997.

Clifton, Daniel, ed. *Chronicle of the 20th Century*. London: Dorling Kindersley, 1995.

Doka, Kenneth J., and Joyce D. Davidson, eds. *Living with Grief: Who We Are, How We Grieve*. Philadelphia: Brunner-Mazel, 1998.

273

Dossey, Larry. *Meaning and Medicine: Lessons from a Doctor's Tales of Breakthrough and Healing*. New York: Bantam Books, 1991.

Eadie, Betty J. *Embraced by the Light*. Placerville, CA: Gold Leaf Press, 1992.

Estés, Clarissa Pinkola. *Women Who Run with the Wolves: Myths and Stories of the Wild Woman Archetype*. New York: Ballantine Books, 1992.

Frankl, Viktor. *Man's Search for Meaning*. New York: Washington Square Press, 1984.

García-Márquez, Gabriel. *One Hundred Years of Solitude*, trans. Gregory Rabassa. New York: Harper and Row, 1970.

Groopman, Jerome. *The Measure of Our Days: New Beginnings at Life's End*. New York: Viking Press, 1997.

Hay, Louise. *You Can Heal Your Life*. Carlsbad, CA: Hay House, 1987.

Hillman, James. *We've Had a Hundred Years of Psychotherapy and the World Is Getting Worse*. New York: HarperCollins, 1993.

_____. *The Soul's Code: In Search of Character and Calling*. New York: Warner Books, 1997.

Keen, Sam. *Fire in the Belly: On Being a Man*. New York: Bantam Books, 1992.

Klein, Allen. *The Courage to Laugh: Humor, Hope, and Healing in the Face of Death and Dying*. New York: J.P. Tarcher/Putnam, 1998.

Kübler-Ross, Elisabeth. *On Death and Dying*. New York: Scribner Classics, 1997.

Lamm, Maurice. *The Jewish Way in Death and Mourning*. New York: Jonathan David Publishers, 1969.

Levine, Stephen. *A Year to Live: How to Live This Year as if It Were Your Last*. New York: Bell Tower (Harmony Books), 1997.

_____. *Who Dies? An Investigation of Conscious Living and Conscious Dying*. Garden City, NY: Anchor Press/Doubleday, 1982.

Longaker, Christine. *Facing Death and Finding Hope*. New York: Doubleday, 1997.

Maclean, Norman. *A River Runs Through It, and Other Stories*. Chicago: University of Chicago Press, 1976.

Meade, Michael. *Men and the Water of Life: Initiation and the Tempering of Men*. San Francisco: HarperSanFrancisco, 1994.

Moore, Thomas. *Care of the Soul: A Guide for Cultivating Depth and Sacredness in Everyday Life*. New York: HarperCollins, 1992.

_____. *The Education of the Heart: Readings and Sources for Care of the Soul, Soul Mates, and the Re-enchantment of Everyday Life*. New York: HarperPerennial, 1996.

Nuland, Sherwin B. *How We Die: Reflections on Life's Final Chapter*. New York: Vintage Books, 1993.

Peck, F. Scott. *Denial of the Soul: Spiritual and Medical Perspectives on Euthanasia*. New York: Harmony Books, 1997.

Pirsig, Robert L. *Zen and the Art of Motorcycle Maintenance*. New York: Bantam New Age Books, 1974.

Raffin, Thomas. "Perspectives on Clinical Medical Ethics." In *Principles of Critical Care*, ed. J. B. Hall, G. R. Schmidt, and L. D. Wood. New York: McGraw-Hill, 1992.

Rapoport, Roger, and Marguerita Castanera, eds. *I Should Have Stayed Home*. Berkeley, CA: Book Passage Press, 1994.

Remen, Rachel. *Kitchen Table Wisdom*. New York: Riverhead Books, 1996.

Rumi, Jelaluddin. *These Branching Moments*, trans. John Moyne and Coleman Barks. Providence, RI: Copper Beech Press, 1988.

Schneiderman, Lawrence, and Nancy Jecker. *Wrong Medicine: Doctors, Patients, and Futile Treatments*. Baltimore: Johns Hopkins University Press, 1995.

Siegel, Bernie. *Love, Medicine and Miracles: Lessons Learned About Self-Healing From a Surgeon's Experience With Exceptional Patients*. New York: Harper and Row Publishers, 1986.

Somé, Malidoma Patrice. *Of Water and the Spirit: Ritual, Magic, and Initiation in the Life of an African Shaman*. New York: Putnam, 1994.

Tatelbaum, Judy. *The Courage to Grieve*. New York: Harper and Row Publishers, 1980.

Terkel, Studs. *The Good War: An Oral History of World War Two*. New York: Pantheon Books, 1984.

Thomas, Lewis. *Lives of the Cell: Notes of a Biology Watcher*. New York: Penguin Books USA, 1995.

Tillich, Paul. *The Courage to Be*. New Haven, CT: Yale University Press, 1952.

Twain, Mark. *The Devil's Racetrack: Mark Twain's Great Dark Writings*. Berkeley, CA: University of California Press, 1966.

Vardey, Lucinda, ed. *God in All Worlds: An Anthology of Contemporary Spiritual Writing*. New York: Vintage Books, 1995.

Webb, Marilyn. *The Good Death: The New American Search to Reshape the End of Life*. New York: Bantam Books, 1997.

Weiss, Brian. *Many Lives, Many Masters*. New York: Simon and Schuster, 1988.

_____. *Only Love Is Real: A Story of Soulmates Reunited*. New York: Warner Books, 1996.

Zimmer, Heinrich: *The King and the Corpse: Tales of the Soul's Conquest of Evil*. Princeton, NJ: Princeton University Press, 1948.

Source Notes

Form 4.1. Copyright California Medical Association 1996. Published with permission of and by arrangement with the California Medical Association. Copies of this form, as well as an accompanying brochure and wallet card, may be obtained from CMA Publications at 800-882-1-CMA.

Form 4.2. Published with permission of and by arrangement with the California Medical Association. Copies of this form may be obtained from CMA Publications at 800-882-1-CMA.

Form 4.3. Copyright M. Brod, et al., 1990, Center for Clinical and Aging Services Research, 3330 Geary Blvd., 2nd Floor, San Francisco, CA 94118.

Form 4.5. Used with permission from St. Joseph Health System, Orange, CA.

Form 4.6. Copyright Commission on Aging with Dignity. To order a copy of "Five Wishes" write to: Aging with Dignity, PO Box 1661, Tallahassee, FL 32302-1661, or visit their web site www.agingwithdignity.org.

The following publishers have given permission to use quotations from copyrighted works:

The True Work of Dying: A Practical and Compassionate Guide to Easing the Dying Process, Jan Bernard and Miriam Schneider. New York: Avon Books, 1996.

Care of the Soul: A Guide for Cultivating Depth and Sacredness in Everyday Life, Thomas Moore. New York: HarperCollins, 1992.

Man's Search For Meaning, Viktor E. Frankl. Boston: Beacon Press, 1992.

Close to the Bone: Life-Threatening Illness and the Search for Meaning, by Jean Shinoda-Bolen. New York: Scribner, 1996.

Index

abandonment, 230
acceptance, 107, 109–10, 111, 120–21
　cure and, 141
　personal, 244
　of soul's needs and messages, 136
　as stage of grief, 153
acupuncture, 120, 175
adolescence, 114
Advance Directives, 27, 27–34
　development of, 115
　as discussion promoters, 30
　evaluations of, 32–33, 35–36
　forms, 36–56
　gaps in, 193
　hypothetical situations in, 23, 30
　invitation to use, 77–78
　obtaining forms/information, 34
　purposes of, 209
　unknowns and, 21–22
afterlife, 110, 211
age, 77
AIDS, 127–29, 134, 141
Allende, Isabel, 157
allies, 184
alternative treatments, 120
Americans with Disabilities Act, 92,
　230

anger, 6, 111
　bodily location of, 178
　re conflicts, 91
　expressing, 168
　at illness, 136, 257
　at patients, 116
　as stage of grief, 153
appreciation, 67
autonomy, 89, 192, 194
　as barrier to connection, 247
　denial of, 208
　respect for, 114

balance, 140
bargaining, 6, 111
　re conflicts, 90
　re illness, 136
　re medical care, 116
　as stage of grief, 153
　upholding, 141
Bartlow, Joshua Fischer, 234, 235
Bartlow, Maya Fischer, 234–35
beneficence, 89–90, 193, 194
Bernadin, Cardinal, 19
Bernard, Jan, 199, 211, 220, 233
birth, 196–97, 234
blame, 124–25, 126–30, 169, 181, 262

personal, 135
    societal, 129
Bly, Robert, 198
body, 173–74
    as energy network, 175
    escaping, 217
    as machine, 174
body language, 75
Bolen, Jean Shinoda, 143, 155, 157
Borges, Jorge Luis, 232
brain injury, 164
Brod, Madlyn, 30

California Living Will, 29
Callahan, Daniel, 59, 89
Campbell, Andrew, 73
cancer, 120
cardiopulmonary resuscitation (CPR),
    24–25, 197, 208
care, 142
caregivers:
    fears, 243
    gifts to, 271
    need for care, 251
    patient's view of, 257–58
    relationship to patients, 114
    separation from patients, 6, 243.
        See also doctors; health care
        providers
Castaneda, Carlos, 184
chakra levels:
    identifying, 100–101
    moving through, 102–4
chakras, 96–97, 98
    higher-level, 99, 100–102. *See also*
        futility
Chatwin, Bruce, 226
children, 62–64, 266
    death of, 61

hero, 71
choice, 120, 121, 134, 169
    all-or-nothing, 145–47 (*see also*
        dichotomies)
    of attitude, 156
    harmful, 132
    illness as manifestation of, 167
Ciofolo, Mary, 185
clinical situation, 23, 28
    Advance Directive application to,
        33
    effect on family members, 69
    health care providers and, 72
comfort care, 91
Commission on Aging with Dignity,
    30, 36
communication, 75–76, 261
    absence of, 8
    bidirectional, 90
    for conflict resolution, 100
    of end-of-life decisions, 18–19
compassion, 67, 158, 214
completion, 256, 265
conferences, family/health care team,
    91–92. *See also* medical ethics
        consultations
conflict resolution, 89–92, 100, 142
conflicts, 18
    ethical, 88–92
    re futility, 94
    level of argument, 93
    participant identification, 100
connection, 118, 210, 217, 239,
    246–47, 267
    of individual, 172
Conrad, Joseph, 202
consciousness, 132
    impairing, 216–17, 265
consent, 192

informed, 90, 113
contradictions, 219
control, 96, 205, 263
    loss of, 246. *See also* power
Cost Containment Committee, 92
cure, 108, 142
    emotions and, 179
    illusion of, 139
    life changes and, 141
curiosity, 143, 144

death:
    acceptance of, 200
    acknowledgment of, 8
    aftermath of, 237
    of children, 61
    communal rituals of, 146
    control of, 120
    denial of, 22
    deserving, 124–25
    as end, 208
    experience of, 3–4
    good, 30, 147–48
    healing via, 264
    historical attitudes toward, 109
    lessons of, 148, 246
    messages of, 221
    modern approach to, 5, 209
    others' preparation for, 157
    preparation for, 255–56
    process of, 233
    stages of, 111–12
    as teacher, 218. *See also* end of life;
        mortality
decision making, 57–59, 193, 195
    control in, 96
    doctors' influence in, 91
    at end of life, 17–19
    guidelines, 83–84

institutional, 59
    participants in, 66
    right to, 97
decisions, 31. *See also* Advance
    Directives
dementia, 132
denial, 18, 111
    of autonomy, 208
    of conflicts, 90
    of death, 22, 112
    of illness, 136
    of shadow, 201, 202, 232
    of soul, 6, 233
    as stage of grief, 153
    of vulnerability, 129, 130
depression, 6, 108, 111
    re illness, 136
    as part of healing, 152
    in relation to medical care, 118–19
    re remission/change, 171
    as stage of grief, 153, 155–56
    work of, 178
descent, 108, 142, 144, 152–60, 186
diagnosis-related groups (DRGs), 117
dichotomies, 108, 125–26, 145–46,
        147, 159–60
discussions, 18–19, 21–25
    Advance Directives and, 30–31
    end of life (*see* end-of-life
        discussions)
    with surrogates, 29
Do Not Resuscitate (DNR) orders, 29
doctors:
    as decision makers, 29
    distrust of, 116
    end-of-life discussions by, 18, 22
    guilt and, 135
    influence on patient, 91
    intent of, 89–90

in medical business, 117–18
mistakes by, 207–8
patients' wishes and, 8
refusal of Advance Directive
    discussions, 78. *See also*
    caregivers; health care providers
documentation, 27
Dossey, Larry, 134, 174
DNR. *See* Do Not Resuscitate orders
dreams, 185
DRGs. *See* diagnosis-related groups
Durable Power of Attorney for Health
    Care Decisions, 29, 32, 33, 35,
    37–39
Dying Well, 30, 32, 33, 36, 46–47, 74

economics, 58
education, 189
elderly, 127, 131
elders, 61–62, 64
emotion, 236–37
    effect on body/illness, 169, 179–80
    rejection of, 245
empathy, 67, 91
emptiness, 201
end of life:
    abuse of, 16
    arranging, 15–19
    children and, 63–64
    conflicts during, 88–89
    desires for, 258–60
    experience of, 63, 217–18
    lessons of, 239
    making futile, 228
    others' role in, 184
    participants in, 57–74, 85, 88, 198
    physical environment for, 235
    planning, 17–19, 21
    purposes of, 31
    qualities for, 147–48

setting for, 88, 163
tasks of, 199–200. *See also* death;
    mortality
end-of-life discussions, 18–19, 21–25,
    76–77
    basic elements of, 77–78
    fear and, 78
    issues in, 100
    sample scenarios, 77–84
energy, 175–76
energy centers. *See* chakras
equality, 192
Ereshkigal, 133, 157, 200
Espinosa, Ernesto, 10
eternal, the, 87, 190, 210–11
    exploration of, 200
ethical responsibilities, 85–88
ethics, 192. *See also* medical ethics
ethics committees, 89, 92
eugenics, 17
euthanasia, 172, 218
evil, admitting, 185
experience, 212
    of death/end of life, 3–4, 63,
    217–18
    evading, 247
    of mysteries, 19
    near-death, 197, 210–11
    sharing, 261
    of soul, 211–12

fairy tales, 139–40, 185
families, 57, 60–62, 69, 70
    burden of illness, 70, 170–71
    goals of, 68–69
    hopes of, 69
    relationships, 85
    responsibility to patient, 89
    role during death process, 9, 91–92
fears, 4, 5, 18, 23, 28, 146

Advance Directive application to, 33
in end-of-life discussions, 78
of family members, 69
of health care providers/caregivers, 71, 89, 243
of mortality, 78, 243
as obstacle, 151–52
fiber, 127
Five Wishes, 30, 32, 33, 36, 48–56
forgiveness, 216, 224, 239
Frankl, Viktor, 109, 142–43, 153, 156, 158–59, 164
friends, 57, 62
futility, 59, 93–96, 116, 227–28
chakra level of discussion re, 96–100

Gabrukeiwicz, Thom, 250
genetic disposition, 127
gifts, 232, 271
effects of, 231–32
receiving, 248
goals, 22, 28, 120
Advance Directive application to, 33
attainment likelihood, 93
defining, 93, 94–95
differing, 94
for end-of-life participants, 67–74
family members', 68–69
health care providers', 71
of soul, 184
God, persons taking role of, 65
God's will, 59
Gould, Stephen Jay, 174
grandparents, 61
grief, 108, 152
aftermath of, 160
anticipatory, 157
completing, 237

final, 258
stages of, 152–53
grieving, 8, 238
Groopman, Jerome, 171
growth, spiritual, 211

harm, 10
Hay, Louise, 179, 181
healers, 109–10
guise of, 113, 114
souls of, 120
task of, 163
wounding by, 180. *See also* care-givers; doctors; health care providers
healing:
ancient wounds, 182–83
death and, 264
depression and, 152
energy and, 176
of health care providers, 258
need for, 18
societal context of, 170
by soul, 271
spiritual elements in, 109
spiritual needs, 10
transformation of, 142
what is needed for, 137
health care, 193, 195
health care providers, 71
choice of role, 247
as decision makers, 89
futility decisions and, 94
healing of, 258
knowledge of patient, 192–93
lack of training, 31
legal responsibilities, 58
patient demands on, 213
patients' effects on, 234, 245
relationship to families, 85

relationship to institutions, 87–88
relationship to patients, 87, 166
roles, 64–67, 216, 220–21. *See also*
    caregivers; doctors; healers;
    nurses
health care system's approach to
    death, 5
heart disease, factors in, 126
Heisenberg, Werner, 174
helplessness, 154
herbs, 177
Hillman, James, 170, 183, 184, 189,
    197
Hippocratic oath, 10, 208
HMOs, 117, 119
home, 260, 261
homeopathy, 177
honesty, 234, 261
hopelessness, 6
hopes, 18, 22, 28
    Advance Directive application to,
        33
    of family members, 69
    of health care providers, 71
    for remainder of life, 22–23
hospice, 88
hospitals, 8, 9, 244–45
humility, 67
humor, 143, 144, 187–88, 259

illness, 196
    blame for, 126 (*see also* blame)
    causes of, 89
    as chemical imbalances, 177
    clinical situation (*see* clinical
        situation)
    context of, 214, 215
    denial of, 136
    deserving, 134
    effect on health care providers,
        73–74

evading, 107
gifts of, 107
iatrogenic, 180
as impetus from soul, 178
meaning of, 129, 134, 142, 174–75
messages of, 25, 170, 181, 217, 221
self-induced, 136, 167–70
as shamanic journey, 186
socially induced, 170
society's response to, 123
spiritual, 171–72
status and, 129
as teacher, 218
terminal, 29
tragedy of, 107
illusions, 220–21
    of cure, 139
    lack of, 159
    loss of, 154, 172–73
    of self, 256
Inanna, 155–56, 157
income, 16
individual, 57, 58, 210
    concept of, 191–92
    connections, 172
    essence of, 142
    honoring, 232, 240
    responsibilities to society, 85
    rights of, 92
    uniqueness of, 198–99
infanticide, 128
infections, 127
information:
    access to, 91
    factual bases of opinions, 100
    re recommendation bases, 95
institutions, 87–88. *See also* hospitals
insurance, 130
intent, 175
    of giving, 231–32
intercession, 110–11

interventions:
    alternatives, 146–48
    benefits/burdens of, 24–25, 28, 33,
        70, 72–74
    investment in, 130
    nursing, 91
    refusal of, 29, 114
    resuscitation, 208, 209
    risk/benefit ratio, 146
    yield/risk ratio, 90
isolation, 146, 152, 219
    of caregiver, 243
    in hospitals, 244
    leaving, 166
    from self, 172

Jecker, Nancy, 93
Joint Commission on Accreditation of
        Healthcare Organizations, 27
judge, 64
judgments, 108, 125, 126, 192
    projection of, 94
    value, 134. *See also* blame
Jung, Carl, 200

karma, 182–83
Kübler-Ross, Elizabeth, 111, 120, 152,
        234

Lamm, Maurice, 196
law, 97
lawsuits, 116
learning, 76
    by soul, 218, 267
legacies, 19, 22, 166, 225–41
    accepting, 238–39
    affirming, 70
    creating, 186–87
    memories as, 257
    midwiving, 233–35
    shaping, 88

    in stories, 262
    time to complete, 220
    written, 30
Levine, Stephen, 141, 157, 190, 199,
        225
liabilities, 97
life:
    end of (*see* end of life; *see also* death)
    honoring, 199
    meanings of, 4 (*see also* meaning)
    moral responsibility to sustain, 70,
        84
    prolonging, 17, 107, 108, 125, 164,
        209
    purposes of, 107
    respect for, 200
    spiritual dimension of, 88
    as test, 214, 216
    value of, 16–17, 22
life after death, 110, 211
life, quality of. *See* quality of life
life support, withdrawal of, 84
lifestyle, 89, 124
listening, 75–76, 91, 190, 214, 234
lives, worth of, 16–17, 22
locked-in state, 164
lodges, 65–66, 88, 92
losses, 159, 263
love, 10, 158, 261
    of self, 183
    sharing, 265–66

Maclean, Norman, 107
maleness, 127
malpractice, 116
Márquez, Gabriel García, 203
meaning, 4, 109, 120, 235–36
    deciphering, 140
    discovery of, 263
    of illness, 129, 134, 142, 174–75
    lack of, 174

yearning for, 227
Medicaid, 117, 130
medical care, 7–8
  as business, 116–18
  defensive, 116
  denial of, 192
  destructiveness of, 5, 9
  prevention of death, 209
  technologic, 15 (*see also*
    technology). *See also*
    interventions
medical ethics:
  focus of, 90
  issues in, 92
  law and, 97
  patient-centered, 193, 194
medical ethics consultations, 96, 97,
    100
  sample, 103–4
Medicare, 117
Meese, Ken, 30, 36, 74
memories, 229, 257
  creative, 236. *See also* legacies
messages:
  of death, 221
  of illness, 25, 170, 181, 217, 221
  interpreting, 184–90
  opening to, 187
  of soul, 136
metaphor, 180, 181
mind, 175
minyans, 66, 92
Mirror Game, 94, 99–100
misunderstanding, 76
Moore, Thomas, 77, 142, 154, 156,
    171, 173, 178, 183
  on religion, 188
morality tales, 226
mortality:
  acknowledgment of, 8, 17, 258, 259
  denial of, 22, 112

fear of, 78, 243. *See also* death; end
    of life
"My Desires for the Last of My Life,"
    28, 30, 36, 45
mysteries, 77, 160
  experience of, 19
Natural Death Act form, 29, 32, 33,
    35, 40–41
near-death experiences, 197, 210–11
needs, 217
  expression of, 88
  patient's, 217, 248
  of soul, 22, 136, 163
  spiritual, 10
Ninshubur, 157
nonmaleficence, 90, 193, 194
nurses, 62, 72, 91, 244. *See also* care-
    givers; health care providers

observation, 174
organs, 178–79
Out of Hospital DNR orders, 29
outcome-based reporting, 67

pain, 190
  avoidance of, 157
  controlling, 216
  existential, 216
  sharing, 158
  as teacher, 218
Pascal's wager, 214
past lives. *See* reincarnation
paternalism, 116, 193, 194
patience, 67
patient's wishes, 8, 113
  expression of, 256 (*see also* Advance
    Directives)
  overriding/superseding, 59, 97
patients:
  as decision makers, 57, 58, 60
  knowledge about, 192–93

meaning to society, 123
needs, 217, 248
relationship to caregivers, 6, 87, 114, 166, 213, 243, 257–58
relationships, 85–88
role in illness, 114
as teachers, 249
values of, 193, 194
patriarch, 65
peace, 109
Peck, Scott, 155, 172, 178, 190, 218
Pinto, Santan, 199
placebo effect, 177
pleasure, 173, 268
power, 89
lack of, 119, 154
loss of, 263–64. *See also* control
power struggles, 94, 97, 99, 228
powers of attorney, 29. *See also* Durable Power of Attorney for Health Care Decisions
presumptions, 174
professionalism, 245
profit, 117, 119
protection, 228
psychology, 182
purposes, 120, 174, 175, 236
of end of life, 31
of life, 107
of soul, 68, 112, 256

quality of life, 22, 23, 28
acceptable, 31
Advance Directive application to, 33
family members', 69
forms re, 29
health care providers', 72
life's value and, 131
Quality of Life Advance Directive, 30, 32, 33, 35, 42–44

quantification, 118, 146
questions:
Advance Directive discussions of, 30–31
re Advance Directives, 28
choice of, 174
re death, 110
for end of life, 9, 18
eternal, 109, 120, 121
evading, 9–10
re purpose, 108
of soul, 250
"what if," 76

rationality, 88, 94
reasons, 132–33
for suffering, 156, 158. *See also* meaning
recommendations, 95
redemption stories, 185–86
reincarnation, 166, 182, 213
relationships, 85–88
religion, 188–90, 200, 210, 211
Remen, Rachel, 245
reorganization, 153
resolution, 153. *See also* acceptance
resource allocation, 15–16, 87, 90
desert and, 130
factors in, 230
value judgments in, 134
resource management, 116
resources, misuse of, 17
responsibilities, 85–88, 115, 135, 192
societal, 89, 90
resuscitation, refusal of, 29. *See also* cardiopulmonary resuscitation
retribution, 130–32
right to die, 115, 209
rights:
individual, 92
losing, 132

risk management, 92
risk managers, 91
Rumi, Jelaluddin, 212

Sagan, Carl, 197, 211, 245
Salk, Jonas, 112
salt, 127
satisfaction, 224
Schneider, Miriam, 199, 211, 220
Schneiderman, Lawrence, 93
science, 174, 210
secular materialism, 214
self-examination, 155
shadow, 200–203, 247
    denial of, 201, 202, 232
shamans' role, 109
shock, 153
siblings, 61
silence, 76, 144, 146
smoking, 127
society, 85
    responsibilities of, 89, 90
Somé, Malidoma, 61
songs, 226
soul, 3, 188–89
    communication by, 76
    as decision maker, 59
    demands of, 247
    denial/evasion of, 5–6, 233
    desires of, 215
    discovery of, 221
    as element in medical care, 109
    eternal, 165, 210
    existence of, 210, 214
    experience of, 211–12
    expression of needs, 88
    finding, 25
    goals of, 184
    healing by, 271
    interpreting messages of, 178,
        184–90

issues of, 101
learning by, 218, 267
manifestations of, 165–66
needs of, 22, 136, 163
neglect of, 169, 172
as *One*, 244, 251, 252
progress of, 196–98
purposes of, 68, 112, 256
secular view of, 146
of society, 123
technology's ignoring of, 112, 113,
    118
treatment of, 164, 218
universal, 166
work of, 149, 163, 172, 213, 217,
    250
spirit, 189
spiritual dimension of life, 88
spiritual exploration, 124
spirituality, 199
Statement of Preferences, 29
stories, 226–27, 262
    creating, 232, 235–37
    honoring, 229
suffering, 153, 172
    costs of, 90
    from medical care, 209–10
    prolonging, 29
    reasons for, 155, 158–59
surrogates, 29, 60

tasks:
    completion of, 256
    pre-death, 142
Tatelbaum, Judy, 152
technology, 111
    prolonging life with, 107, 108, 125,
        164, 209
    as sole care method, 149
    stages of, 112–21
    wounding by, 119

therapy, benefits of, 24–25, 28, 33
  to family members, 70
  to health care providers, 73–74
therapy, burdens of, 24, 28, 33
  on family members, 70
  on health care providers, 72–73
Tillich, Paul, 183
time, 199, 260
touch, 148, 260
treatment alternatives, 15–16. *See also*
  interventions
trust, 267
truth, 174
Tucker, Beatrice, 212

understanding, 5, 91, 158
  practices for, 220
unknowns, 21
utilization review, 92

values, 18, 90
  family, 126
  of the nonquantifiable, 16–17, 22,
    146

  patient's, 193, 194
  societal, 87
  stating, 29
victimization, 170
vision quest, 186–87

war, 112, 113
waste, 133
Weiss, Brian, 182, 213
wholeness, 6
wisdom, sources of, 10
wishes, statements of, 27. *See also*
    Advance Directives; patient's
    wishes
witnesses, 67, 89
work, 125
Wrong Medicine, 93

Young, Ernlé, 228
youth, 114
  ignoring, 134
  right to care, 131

Zimmer, Heinrich, 185

About the Author

Bruce G. Bartlow, M.D., has been practicing medicine for more than twenty-five years, mostly in San Francisco and surrounding areas. Board certified in internal medicine, nephrology and critical care, he has been on staff at several hospitals, including Mt. Zion and St. Luke's in San Francisco. He now practices critical care, nephrology and ethics in Redding, California.